THIS BOOK BELONGS TO

The Library of

....

....

@COPYRIGHT 2024

Did you like my book? I pondered it severely before releasing this book. Although the response has been overwhelming, it is always pleasing to see, read or hear a new comment. Thank you for reading this and I would love to hear your honest opinion about it. Furthermore, many people are searching for a unique book, and your feedback will help me gather the right books for my reading audience.

Thanks!

Table of Contents

INTRODUCTION

Cannabis is used as a drug, as an affiliate intoxicant, and as a religious ritual. Significant pharmaceutical companies were around before cannabis was available under the Marijuana Tax Act of 1937. Provided medicines for cannabis. By the mid-20th century, the perception of cannabis and its components had shifted from frequently prescribed medical therapy to dangerous narcotics, fueled by concerns of enhanced recreation and incomplete knowledge of how cannabis operates within the body. The prohibition of cannabis was motivated more by social stresses and baseless worries than by real scientific evidence of the medicinal value of the drug.

You've likely learned about the three-letter CBD buzzword at this stage at the moment. More people than ever turn to this organic and natural remedy for a variety of reasons. They are many variables that contribute to CBD's increasing popularity. One of them is legalization in some areas of the United States (and some nations around the globe). Another factor is the growing amount of studies that demonstrate the different medical advantages of CBD.

But what's the CDB? If you're a newbie in the CBD globe and you're interested in learning more about this item, then you've come to the correct location. In this post, we will present you to a fantastic compound called CBD.

Was this decrease in the notoriety of cannabis as a medicine overturned at the start of the 1960s? When Dr. Raphael Mechoulam, a Bulgarian / Israeli natural goods scientist, first discovered the composition of THC, the main psychoactive component of cannabis.

Mechoulam and his crew at the Hebrew University moved on to uncover the human endocannabinoid system, the physiological structure within the body accountable for intercellular signaling, and the extensive regulation of appetite and metabolism. The impacts of cannabis stem from its contact with the endocannabinoid system.

The human body produces products called cannabinoids or endocannabinoids. Endocannabinoids stimulate cell membrane receptors throughout the body, particularly within the brain and intestines. There are three main kinds of cannabinoids: endocannabinoids, phytocannabinoids (such as cannabis-based THC) and synthesized cannabinoids such asHU-210 created by Mechoulam's group (HU stands for Hebrew University) that are a powerful pain reliever and prospective Alzheimer's therapy.

In the 1990s, cannabis was shown to provide relief from the kinds of pain that morphine-type drugs could not cause (Russo in Pain Management, 2001). Cannabis was also one of the few drugs that could avoid or inverse waste syndrome in cancer and AIDS patients (Gorter in Cancer, Cachexia, and Cannabinoids, 2000). These insights into the body's endocannabinoid system have merged to further the rehabilitation of cannabis as modern medicine.

CANNABIS EXPLAINED: WHAT IS IT AND WHAT CAN IT DO FOR YOU?

Cannabis, additionally stated as marijuana could be a mind-altering drug used for medical or recreational functions within the Cannabis plant. The first psychedelic portion of cannabis is psychoactive substance (THC), one amongst 483 cannabis compounds recognized within the plant, as well as a minimum of sixty-five alternative cannabis compounds. Cannabinoids. Cannabis may be used for smoking, spraying or in meat or as an extract.

Cannabis has a mental and physical impact, such as generating "high" or "stoned" impressions, a particular shift in perception, an improvement in mood, and an increase in appetite. Effects are measured in minutes when smoked, and in about 30 to 60 minutes when fried and consumed. The impact lasts between two and six hours. Short-term facet effects might embrace memory loss, dry mouth, impaired motor skills, red eyes, and psychosis or anxiety. Long-term side effects may include addiction, and reduced cognitive ability Short-term facet effects might embrace memory loss, dry mouth, impaired motor skills, red eyes, and psychosis or anxiety long adolescents, and cognitive problems in children whose parents used cannabis during pregnancy. There is an active link between cannabis use and the risk of psychosis, although the cause-and-effect discussion is that marijuana is commonly used for cannabis use. Recreation or as a medicinal product, although it may also be used for spiritual purposes. In 2013, between 128 and 232 million individuals used cannabis (2.7% to 4.9% of the world's inhabitants between 15 years of era) is the most widely used illicit drug in both the world and the United States, although it is also legal. In some jurisdictions. Zambia, the United States, Canada, and Nigeria are the countries with the most exceptional adult use as of 2018. Some call it to weed, some cal it pot, others call it marijuana.

As weeds become legal in more fields, names for plants are developing. Today, more and more individuals use the word cannabis to refer to weed. Some claim that this is a correct name. Others think it is more benign, as opposed to words like weed or pot, which some individuals still identify with its illegal use.

Cannabis is generally used for its soothing and relaxing impacts. In some U.S. states, it is also prescribed to assist with a variety of medical circumstances, including chronic pain, glaucoma, and poor appetite.

Keep in mind that while cannabis derives from a plant and is considered natural, it can still have strong positive and harmful effects.

WHAT CBD IS AND HOW IT IS MADE

CBD

CBD is a phytochemical–a plant-based compound. It's been storming the medical and wellness world over the last century. CBD originates from a cannabis plant, frequently referred to as hemp in English.

CBD does interact with the endocannabinoid system. It is a network of receptor nerves shared by the vast majority of animal communities, from insects to reptiles, people, and domestic animals. The reality that the variety of animal species is distributed demonstrates that the endocannabinoid system has likely developed over millions of years earlier. It is essential to the working of the human body.

CBD appears to reduce swelling–leading, among other variables, to pain relief. It has also been engaged in the battle against anxiety, depression, rheumatoid arthritis, stress, and dozens of other problems that people face periodically.

Hemp

Hemp has been used for its crops, fibers, and medicinal products for millennia. CBD occurs in relatively large quantities in the leaves, seeds, and flowers of the hemp plant. CBD had to work its advantages on the consumers of hemp long before we learned anything about the molecule itself.

CBD is a suite of cannabinoids. These are the chemicals that best communicate with the endocannabinoid system. They are generated in small amounts by some species of black truffle and echinacea, but mainly by cannabis.

Cannabinoids are believed to be accountable for defending cannabis crops from sun damage to UV rays. Plants are also considered to safeguard against insect grazing. The adhesive nature of the cannabinoid cocktail implies that it sticks in the mouths of the insects who are trying to consume the plant. Terpenes and flavonoids found alongside cannabinoids have an overpowering taste, which also adds to defense against insects.

How It Is Extracted

There are numerous products produced with CBD: gummy bears, infused water, tablets, steam oil, tinctures, and others. Despite this, there are still only three main methods to extract CBD from the cannabis crop: the production of alcohol, oil, and supercritical CO_2.

Alcohol removal includes steeping the leaves, branches, and flower sections of the hemp plant in a high-alcohol solution or pure alcohol. The blend is boiled, and the entire spectrum of cannabinoids is leaked out of the plant material and into the liquid. This is an inexpensive and comparatively easy technique.

The removal of oil functions in a comparable manner to the production of alcohol. Plant sections wealthy in CBD are entirely immersed in liquid, this time in edible oil. The oil may be olive, coconut, grape seed, or several others. Again, as in the case of alcohol production, oil extraction produces a complete spectrum of cannabinoid compounds and is simple to do and cheap.

Supercritical CO_2

The art of supercritical CO2 extraction of CBD has been perfected by a tiny amount of businesses in the latest years. CO2 is carbon dioxide, a prevalent gas in the atmosphere. CO2 is wholly heated and then used to remove the CBD from the plant material. This technique is expensive and complicated, but it enables these companies to generate up to 99 percent pure CBD.

Things CBD Will Do For Your Health

The health blessings of marijuana can not be over-emphasized. In specific, the compound cannabidiol, aka CBD, is increasingly being researched for the leadership of certain health circumstances, and the medical community is More involvement in the option of a non-psychoactive compound. After it soared in popularity last year, too, the overall public is getting more enthusiastic about how CBD can be useful for you, from anxiety control to its anti-inflammatory characteristics, and so much more.

But while CBD is a compelling drug for a slew of health and wellness advantages, it's certainly not a remedy for everything. While there is no denying that CBD can relieve symptoms related to a range of physical and mental health issues, it can not fully heal severe illnesses, as some may argue. Because CBD I such a popular subject right now, it can be hard to distinguish facts from myths. However, as with any other drug or medicine, it's essential to look at what science says when it comes to finding out if it can help you.

So, what does CBD do for your health?

Here are five medical issues that CBD has shown can help with

CBD Can Reduce Anxiety

Although the study is regulated, NPR recorded trials in both livestock and humans indicate that CBD is an anxiolytic. Placed, it can decrease your anxiety. Elisabeth Mack, RN, CEO, and founder of Holistic Caring, says to Bustle, "CBD helps to reduce anxiety." CBD Has Neuroprotective Properties Put merely, ingesting CBD on the reg can be useful for your cognitive wellness. "Irrespective of what your specific health needs are, CBD is a neuroprotective agent as well as an antioxidant," studies show that CBD is not only a useful substance When it goes to stopping nerve and brain damage, it can also assist in balancing the signs of degenerative neurological disorders. Try to incorporate CBD coffee into your daily routine to get the brain-boosting advantages of this cannabis compound.

CBD will facilitate Sleep

Problems analysis on the effectuality of CBD in sleep disorder has shown that the substance has the potential to treat bound sleep disorders. There is, however, a tiny catch: Mack says, depending on the individual, that some truly feel energized by CBD. So, eating a few CBD-infused gums in the AM may be more conducive to your sleep-wake cycle, "I advise individuals to carry CBD during the day and see," she suggests.

CBD Can Help Reduce Chronic Pain

There are well-known trails that demonstrate that CBD is a potent anti-inflammatory drug. "Considering that science is starting to suggest that inflammation may be at the root of many wellness problems, it's no wonder that taking anti-inflammatory drugs such as CBD can decrease pain. Research points out that CBD can assist decrease pain. Otherwise, folks would be prescribed it as a primary line of defense instead of therapy, "she adds," However, it will facilitate heighten therapy, and that they realize that CBD has anti-tumor properties in mice, however, isn't tried to cure cancer. "CBD Can't Stop Alzheimer's Disease Progression Even though CBD has been shown to support brain health, it can not prevent the development of A. Thus neither CBD nor THC can stop the disease from occurring. "Although Alzheimer's Society notes that some study indicates that cannabis compounds can assist patients in handling some of the signs of the disease, it also states that no research has discovered that cannabis compounds can treat it. It's not a side-effect-free substance Like any medicine, and you should consult with your doctor before integrating CBD

CBD for Cancer: Can It Help?

- As cancer treatment
- As complementary treatment
- As a preventive
- Side effects
- Products
- Takeaway

Cannabidiol (CBD) is one of many cannabinoids that can be found in hemp and marijuana, two types of cannabis plants.

CBD may assist cancer patients in handling some of the signs of the disease as well as the side effects of therapy. Scientists are also looking at how CBD can help with cancer treatment, but more study is required before any findings can be drawn.

Marijuana has enough tetrahydrocannabinol (THC) to get you high, but hemp doesn't. CBD itself does not have any psychoactive compounds. CBD products may, however, have trace quantities of THC.

Let's take a more in-depth look at how CBD can assist individuals with cancer.

As A Cancer Treatment

There is definite proof to support the concept that cannabinoids can decrease tumor development in animal cancer systems. CBD may also improve the uptake or potency of certain drugs used to cure cancer.

Here is some successful research: in vitro and in vivo research concentrating on pancreatic cancer have shown that cannabinoids can help slow tumor development, decrease tumor invasion, and cause tumor cell death. The writers of the study stated that there is a lack of and urgent need for investigations into the efficacy of distinct formulations, dosing, and accurate method of operation.

It stated that CBD could cause cell death and render glioblastoma cells more susceptible to radiation, but without having an impact on healthy cells.

A large, long-term study of Men in the California Men's Health Study cohort discovered that cannabis use could be inversely correlated with the danger of bladder cancer. However, a connection between cause and effect has not been created.

A 2014 research in experimental designs of colon cancer in vitro indicates that CBD may prevent the distribution of colorectal cancer bacteria.

A study of 35 in vitro and in vivo research discovered that cannabinoids are promising compounds for the therapy of gliomas.

Another study has shown the efficacy of CBD in pre-clinical designs of metastatic breast cancer. The research discovered that CBD considerably decreased the spread and invasion of breast cancer cells.

These are just a few trials that address the ability of cannabinoids to assist cure cancer. Still, it is far too early to conclude that CBD is a secure and efficient therapy for cancer in animals. CBD should not be regarded as a replacement for other cancer treatments.

Some fields for future studies include: the impacts of CBD with and without other cannabinoids, such as THC, on safe and efficient dosing on the effects of distinct administration techniques on particular kinds of cancer, how CBD interacts with chemotherapy drugs and other cancer treatments Complementary therapy for cancer Cancer treatments, such as chemotherapy and radiation, and CBD is also thought to have anti-inflammatory and anti-anxiety characteristics.

To date, only one CBD drug has been approved by the Food and Drug Administration (FDA) The medicine is Epidiolex, and its only use is in the therapy of two unusual types of epilepsy. No CBD products have been approved by the FDA to cure cancer or signs of disease or to reduce the side effects of cancer treatment.

On the other hand, two marijuana-based drugs have been approved for the treatment of nausea and vomiting caused by chemotherapy. Dronabinol (Marinol) arrives in the shape of a capsule and includes THC. Nabilone (Cesamet) is an oral synthetic cannabinoid comparable to THC.

Nabiximols, another cannabinoid drug, is accessible in Canada and sections of Europe. It is a breath foam comprising both THC and CBD and is promising in the treatment of cancer pain. It is not endorsed in the United States but is the topic of continuing studies.

If you are considering using medical marijuana, speak to your doctor about the best way to administer it. Smoking may not be a healthy option for individuals with certain kinds of cancer.

CBD and other cannabis products come in many types, including vapors, tinctures, sprays, and oils. It may also be discovered in candies, coffee, or other edibles.

As a Cancer Prevention

Studies on the position of cannabinoids in cancer growth Mixed A 2010 survey using a mouse model discovered that cannabinoids could cause immune system repression. This could render consumers more vulnerable to certain kinds of cancer. This specific study engaged in cannabis comprising THC.

CBD study has a long way to go when it comes to cancer prevention. Scientists will need to perform long-term research of individuals using particular CBD products, frequency control, dosing, and other factors.

CBD Side Effects

The World Health Organization (WHO) maintains that CBD has an excellent safety profile and that adverse side effects may be due to relationships with other drugs. It says that there is no proof of public health issues arising from the use of mere CBD.

CBD is usually secure and has few side effects. Among them are: appetite modifications that could be a useful thing for individuals in cancer treatment with diarrhea fatigue weight modifications More study is required to know other impacts of CBD, such as whether it impacts hormones

CBD may interfere with liver enzymes that assist in metabolizing certain drugs. This could contribute to higher levels of these drugs in the environment.

CBD, like grapefruit, interferes with the metabolism of certain drugs. Talk to your doctor before using CBD, particularly if you are taking medication that comes with a "grapefruit alert" or one of the following: antibiotic antidepressants or anti-anxiety medications blood thinners muscle relaxers, sedatives or sleeping aids oral or IV chemotherapy The American Cancer Society promotes the need for further studies on cancer cannabinoids pat.

Choosing CBD products

CBD is a natural substance, but natural elements must also be approached with caution and due diligence.

There's a lot of variability in CBD products. Some labels of CBD products create misleading health allegations.

After evaluating 84 CBD products marketed online, scientists discovered that about 43 percent had a higher level of CBD than indicated. Approximately 26% had less CDB than stated.

If you are presently being handled for cancer, maintain in mind that many drugs may communicate with other therapies. This involves CBD, other cannabinoids, or even nutritional and herbal supplements.

Talk to your doctor about the prospective advantages and hazards of CBD, what to look for, and where to buy it. Here are a few factors to consider when selecting CBD products: Hemp-derived CBD products should have only trace quantities of THC.

Products with marijuana-derived CBD may comprise enough THC to generate elevated levels of THC.

Levitate products that create over-the-top wellness allegations.

Compare tags to see how much CBD genuinely exists in the item.

It may take time to find the optimal dose and feel the effects, so a llttle patience is needed. It's a good idea, to begin with, a tiny dose and gradually boost it.

CBD should not be used instead of other cancer treatments. We need more rigorous studies on the prospective advantages and hazards of CBD, dosing, administration, and how it impacts other cancer therapies.

Currently, there are no FDA-approved cancer CBD products. Thus, apart from Epidiolex for epilepsy, the products accessible have not been assessed by the Agency.

Even so, some individuals are using cannabinoids to reduce the side effects of cancer treatment. Because CBD can communicate with other cancer therapies, it's best to verify with your doctor before you begin taking

The Different Types Of Cbd

The next day we're continuing our search to teach the universe about CBD. If you lost our first blog, All Hemp Is Not Equal, make sure you check it out.

It's time to explain the distinct kinds of CDBs. We've been marked a beauty brand at Kush Queen, but we're always going to be the first and ever the cannabis business. We spent years cultivating, extracting, and teaching as much about the plant as we could.

Our products are intended for self-care and wellness. We were aiming to produce a variety of products that would honor the plant in its most efficient shape to assist you to attain ultimate well-being. In our knowledge, feeding our endocannabinoid system frequently is not only a way to feel better, but also a way to exercise preventive wellness. With that, Being the philosophy that drives us, the sort of CBD is crucial to some customers and, as always, transparency at Kush Queen is our main concern. Consequently, we always mention some CDB in each item. We thoroughly regarded each of the products and the sort of CDB used with you in mind.

Hemp Seed Oil

Hemp Seed oil is hot pushed with hemp plants. It does not involve any CBD or phytocannabinoids.

Isolate

Some products comprise a CBD isolate, a purified CBD molecule. The CBD inhibitor is smooth and powdery in shape. It does not include other phytocannabinoids such as complete or full spectrum.

Full-Spectrum

Full Spectrum relates to cannabis-derived from the whole plant containing CBD and other phytocannabinoids such as THC, CBN, THCA, CBC, and CBG.

Broad-Spectrum

Broad Spectrum includes all plant phytocannabinoids but does not contain any detectable quantity of THC.

Nano CBD

Nano CBD is a compound where CBD molecules are reduced to incredibly tiny dimensions (less than 100 nm) and transformed into a water-based shape. This method enables CBD to move through the skin much more readily and rapidly than any oil-based type.

THE LEGALITY AND HISTORY OF CBD

At the beginning of 1998, the British government authorized a business called GW Pharmaceuticals to grow cannabis and developed an accurate and coherent extract for use in clinical trials. GW co-founder Geoffrey Guy, MD, was persuaded and persuaded the Home Office that GW could create cannabis-based medicines with little or no psychoactive impact by using CBD-rich crops.

That summer at the conference of the International Cannabinoid Research Society (ICRS). Concerning counteract the psychoactivity of THC, Guy said that CBD provided its advantages. GW has acquired its CBD-rich varieties from the genetic library of HortaPharm, a Dutch seed company operated by American expatriate horticulturists David Watson and Henry Martyn Robert Clarke.

CBD-rich cannabis contains a long history of use within the treatment of health issues. Within the nineteenth century, Empress used CBD-rich cannabis for discharge cramps. Animal studies have long advised that CBD decreases anxiety and reduces the seriousness and frequency of seizures. But, until a few years earlier, CBD-rich varieties were usually not accessible to cannabis consumers in California and other regions. Generations of marijuana cultivation for peak THC and high THC decreased CBD to trace quantities in most cannabis strains in Northern California, the American cannabis breadbasket.

Dr. Tod Mikuriya, the founder of the Society of Cannabis Clinicians, articulated his wish that "our Burbanks in the Hills" of Northern

California would produce CBD-rich varieties if and once analytical laboratories began to serve the medical cannabis sector.

As years have passed, additional and more brilliant scientific studies involving CBD are represented at conferences of the ICRS, the International Association for Cannabinoid medication, and Patients Out of your time. Some California physicians held up with the study and O'Shaughnessy commented on it, but we were just spectators, not respondents, until the spring of 2009, when Oakland's Steep Hill Laboratory tried cannabis samples from the Harborside Health Center and discovered a few species with more CBD than THC.

Before long, several dozen medical marijuana laboratories calibrated cannabinoid proportions and identified occasional CBD-rich strains. For information collection reasons, we originally described "CBD-rich" as 4 percent or more of dry weight. About balanced strains with approximately equivalent quantities of CBD and THC, a couple of CBD-dominant twists with a ratio of 20-to-1 CBD: THC or higher have been identified to support the CBD-rich cottage sector, petroleum extracts, and other CBD-rich goods.

CBD has been creating contentious reports in Acadiana and across the state. Legislators are taking measures to potentially alter the legality of CBD products.

There is usually a thought regarding CBD. Unlike THC, it is not about to get you high. While the two originate from the same species, the cannabis plant, the CBD can be obtained from the hemp. That portion is the stem of the plant.

CBD is like a weed without heavy, and those who swear by it claim it helps everything from pain, insomnia, depression, and much more.

According to the Hemp Business Journal, CBD revenues have risen tremendously over the last four years and are anticipated to expand even more by 2022. Everyone, from cannabis manufacturers to hemp farmers, is developing products to satisfy the requirement.

It can be discovered in lotions, bath products, coffee, and dog food. While it can be used in a wide range of products, many still wonder why it is illegal.

What creates embarrassment is that, nationally, it's all right and legal. However, there is no difference in Louisiana between cannabis, hemp, and CBD goods.

The law brings all of them under the same umbrella of narcotics. Under state law, CBD-containing goods are still regarded as narcotics in Schedule 1.

Law-makers are presently contemplating a proposal that would allow producers to develop hemp in the state. That proposal is going through a periodic meeting right now and could explain Louisiana's legal position on the legality of hemp and CBD.

Cannabidiol (CBD) is a phytocannabinoid that was found in 1940 and has a lengthy and wealthy background.

However, since almost 4000 years BCE, beings have been cultivating cannabis, both natural cannabis and industrial hemp used in textiles, paper, and strings. Human development has been floating around cannabis, but the legal and medical use it has seen today is the latest occurrence!

In 1563, the Portuguese doctor Garcia da Orta noted that his employees who had taken marijuana were delighted and very starving. At about the same moment, Chinese doctor Li Shizhen recorded the anti-nausea impacts of cannabis. There was also a tale stating that Queen Victoria used marijuana to relieve her menstrual cramps!

However, the real history of CBD starts in 1940, when the American organic chemist Roger Adams removed the CBD compound without understanding for sure what he had removed.

In 1960, the Israeli organic chemist Raphael Mechoulam was able to separate and define the chemical structure of CBD. The chemists could then verify that CBD was a non-psychoactive cannabis component. By the mid-1970s, British accumulation cited CBD tinctures for medical use.

The medical impacts of CBD were created public in America with the release of Charlotte Figi's tale—a teenage girl's unusual seizure disturbance was handled with powerful CBD therapy. And this story was quickly followed by the fight for the legal CDB.

By the Fifties, CBD had been unlawful altogether fifty states. However, the event of science and medication brought the lawfulness of CBD back to question.

In 2017, the FDA took the primary strides towards the approval of CBD for medical uses, and nowadays it's legal altogether fifty States. It is now well recognized for its capacity to decrease stress and anxiety, alleviate pain, promote sleep, and encourage a better and healthier life.

THE DIFFERENCE BETWEEN CBD AND THC

The primary difference between CBD (cannabidiol) and THC (tetrahydrocannabinol) is that CBD does not cause high concentrations, whereas THC does.

Although CBD and THC share a near-exact molecular formula of C21H30O2 and a molecular weight of 314,469 g / mol and 314,464 g / mol respectively, the compounds respond quite differently.

THC, the psychoactive element of marijuana, induces sleep, or drowsiness (a widespread impact of most marijuana strains), while CBD holds you up and improves energy. And THC is accountable for getting warm or low in the body.

When responding together, CBD effectively operates against the impacts of THC by decreasing anxiety, stress, or other adverse emotions. For this purpose, CBD is often used individually for non-psychoactive (and non-recreational) reasons.

CBD is only one of about 400 compounds in marijuana and is accountable for counteracting the impacts of THC. Although the CBD molecule is almost identical to the THC molecule, it doesn't make you happy. On its own, CBD has been shown to have many health advantages and utilizes, such as anxiety, pressure, epilepsy, and depression. The compound is non-psychoactive, which has helped to obtain assistance for its medicinal characteristics in many therapeutic areas.

Its advantages have been maximized in the retail and recreational industries, with CBD products including oils, vapes, medications, skincare, and beverages. Cannabinoid oil is a natural CBD product. Companies from American Eagle to Ben & Jerry's have announced plans to add CBD to some of their fresh goods.

However, the discussion on its legality continues rather complicated. Marijuana remains a nationally illegal drug, and some countries, such as New York, have tried to break down on the sale of CBD-containing meat and beverage. That said, some states have, on their own, legalized the use of CBD, although these countries have very rigid norms for what medical circumstances they can use to handle.

CBD has also been used in animals to handle circumstances such as anxiety, mobility, discomfort, and heart illness. Products such as dog treatments and oils have become increasingly common in the latest years and are often suggested by veterinary surgeons. Antibiotic characteristics of CBD have also been related to assisting combat infection, although the study is blended.

Side Effects Of CBD

Based on the present studies, the side effects of CBD are somewhat restricted. According to research conducted by Medical Marijuana Inc., some incidents of drowsiness, dry mouth, and low blood pressure have been reported, but no severe side effects have been identified.

What's Up With THC?

THC or tetrahydrocannabinol is a psychoactive element of marijuana, although THC is amazingly comparable to its non-psychoactive counterpart CBD. THC is what makes you young, and is therefore somewhat less approved for medicinal use than CBD.

Still, THC boasts of its beneficial uses. THC has characteristics known to assist manage pain, nausea, asthma, and even anorexia nervosa. As a psychoactive compound, however, its therapeutic purposes are still contentious.

Side Effects Of THC

As a compound in a federally illegal drug, the impacts and advantages of THC research are relatively restricted. However, what study has been undertaken has identified a range of effects from THC.

Common adverse side effects in high THC concentrations include decreased cognitive function, fear, paranoia, dry mouth, red eyes, lethargy, and enhanced appetite. Nevertheless, the beneficial impacts of THC include enhanced relaxation, joint, and headache relief, among others. It is worth noting that the increased appetite impact is often seen as beneficial among chemotherapy clients experiencing severe loss of appetite, as well as people suffering from eating disorders.

Health Benefits Of CBD Vs. THC

The health benefits of CBD have been extensively investigated. With its non-psychoactive status, CBD has been known to handle health issues, especially epilepsy. The United States. The Deputy Commissioner for Food and Drug Administration Anna K. Abram said so much.

"CBD is useful in experimental designs of several neurological disorders, including seizure and epilepsy," Abram stated in a notification to the Federal Register in 2017.

The beneficial advantages of compounds such as CBD are becoming increasingly apparent.

The FDA is conscious that' cannabis or marijuana-derived medicines are used for a variety of medical circumstances, including, for instance, AIDS loss, epilepsy, neuropathic pain, therapy of spasticity connected with multiple sclerosis, and cancer and chemotherapy-induced nausea,' according to their website. However, the use of much medical marijuana and even CBD products is still pending formal permission.

Although not used for as many apps as CBD, THC itself boasts quite a few health advantages. In cannabis-oil type, surveys have shown that THC can be used to cure neurodegenerative illnesses such as Alzheimer's and Parkinson's. These trials have also shown that THC can relieve pain and assist in reducing multiple sclerosis.

CBD vs. THC Anxiety

Both THC and CBD have been used for the treatment of depression.

CBD has been used as an anxiolytic or anxiety-treating drug for some achievement. Studies have shown its ability to cure not only anxiety but also depression, PTSD, and obsessive-compulsive disorder.

However, THC has mixed results when it comes to the treatment of anxiety. Due to its psychoactive nature, THC has been associated with emotions of fear or paranoia (maybe most frequently encountered during marijuana use). However, the amount or quantity of THC current is mainly accountable if the customer feels nervous or not, so the suitable amount is more of the main factor.

Negative Effects

While the jury is still out in some respects, trials have shown comparatively few adverse side effects of CBD and THC use so far. However, some experiments have shown that the neurotransmission mechanisms engaged in the handling of CBD can be related to cannabis addiction and reliance, and have discovered connections to the three phases of addiction. Positive impacts have also been identified in the research.

Besides, the THC compound in marijuana may have different impacts on anxiety stimulation. Various trials have shown enhanced anxiety with marijuana use, but findings differ widely based on the individual's condition of anxiety or paranoia.

Legality Of CBD Vs. THC

The validity of both CBD and THC has been under discussion for quite a while. Apart from the national debate (some may contend globally) on the legalization of marijuana, the health advantages of CBD are still mainly untapped by the FDA rules.

In reality, the Drug Enforcement Administration (DEA) has tried several occasions, more lately in 2016, to identify both THC and CBD as Schedule I drugs under the U.S. Controlled Substances Act means "no presently approved medical use and strong potential for abuse." Despite this opposition, ongoing medical information and studies continue to flood in support of legalizing elements such as CBD for extensive use.

However, as of the publication of this paper, CBD is illegal in all 50 States. Although the 2014 Farm Bill semi-legalized production of hemp, it only covered a small set of opportunities for the cultivation of hemp, such as academic and research purposes.

THC is often looped in legal marijuana. As of 2018, medical cannabis is legal in 28 countries plus Washington, D.C. However, the legality of the purchase or use of THC is still somewhat convoluted approximately only for states that have already created medicinal or recreational cannabis legal.

Although a lot fuzzy, it is intelligent to be careful when buying or using CBD products, as their legality is still dubious. The same applies to THC, which is perhaps the most contentious compound of both for legal use.

CBD Investment Opportunity CBD has been used for beverage oil products, but most lately, it is an epilepsy drug called Epidiolex, pending permission by the FDA. If consent is acquired, the over $1 billion marijuana sector could have an enormous investment opportunity. Several businesses have started purchasing cannabis manufacturers in anticipation, particularly Scott's Miracle-Gro Co.

The decision on the authorization of Epidiolex by the FDA and the use of CBD in such drugs is laid for the beginning of June. Not only do we see a rise in the legalization of marijuana, but the recreational advantages of compounds contained in a pot, such as CBD, have an enormous market and investment capacity.

Increased legalization of marijuana Recreational and medical marijuana has seen a considerable increase in approval ratings in recent years, according to Gallup's surveys. With more and more countries legalizing its use, both THC and CBD have the capacity for recreational and manufacturing apps. And, with the enormous market for marijuana willing to be tapped, we should see higher opportunities for investment in CBD-related manufacturing.

Currently, there are a series of countries that have adopted the full legalization of both medical and recreational marijuana, the most recent being Illinois. There is a noticeable rise from just 4-5 years earlier. Twenty-two other countries have enacted legislation enabling medical marijuana under certain circumstances, while several other states have restricted medical CBD allowances if the person meets specific requirements.

For now, it is essential to understand the distinction between CBD and THC as the legalization of medical marijuana is becoming increasingly successful.

VARIOUS FORMS OF CBD AND THC: HOW IS IT DISTRIBUTED ON THE MARKET?

These conditions apply to the composition of cannabinoids in the item, of which CBD is only one (THC being the most well-known), and each possibly having its effect on the endocannabinoid receptor structures discovered throughout the human body. The full-spectrum tag shows that 100 percent of the 100 + cannabinoids in the plant have been removed and are present in the item, including THC at or below 0.3 percent. You may opt for such a formula if you are expecting to accomplish the Entourage Effect, a phenomenon that suggests that a substantial spectrum of compounds interacting with each other can have an effect on your chemistry on the overall impacts of the item.

On the other side, an onion, which is the type of CBD used in our Standard Dose Tincture, is the purest type of the compound because it has been fully obtained from other cannabinoids and plant components, including terpenes and flavonoids. It is tasteless and odorless and can ingest in a variety of ways, including high doses, without the risk of intoxication. When it is to accurate dosing, the isolates are the most reliable because they constitute the quantity of CBD present by amount. They have no flavor or smell and are an excellent way to go if you're looking for anti-inflammatory characteristics because you're not subjected to THC.

Large-spectrum products, comprising the full spectrum of cannabinoids except for THC, are falling somewhere in the center area. This implies that you can experiment with the consequences of mixing various compounds (the Entourage Effect) while still abstaining from the psychoactive effects of THC. It is useful to note that study into the impacts of cannabinoids beyond CBD is changing the industry in real-time as we know about the incredibly complicated endocannabinoid system.

The THC shapes. Does that imply that the other types are not marijuana?

Marijuana study is just beginning to touch the surface of the hundred-plus cannabinoids discovered inside the trichomes of the plant. These cannabinoids include various forms of THC and CBD, lesser-known cannabinoids such as sleep-inducing cannabinol (CBN) and anti-bacterial cannabigerol (CBG), and some that we don't hear about yet. Although pharmaceutical companies have created synthetic THC types, everything you see for purchase at a dispensary is plant-derived.

THC is such a famous cannabinoid that some individuals are wearing it on their backs.

THC is such a famous cannabinoid that some individuals carry it on their chests. Piccadilly-dependents Tetrahydrocannabinol (THC) is the most prevalent and well-known cannabinoid in most psychoactive marijuana crops. The bulk of THC in marijuana crops is an acidic type of THC called THCA that is only psychoactive when triggered by heat, which causes THCA to periodic, trippy THC. Commercial extractors are beginning to experiment with Delta-8-THC, another type of cannabinoid that is useful for the treatment of nausea and eating diseases, while 11-Hydroxy-THC is a dominant, metabolized type of THC that your body produces orally after consuming marijuana, which is why edibles may seem overpowering even if you are a standard toker.

Qualities of each Isolate Tasteless and odorless contribute to any beverage or plate without influencing taste No danger of exposure to THC Multi-format supply may be administered topically as a salve, sublingually as a tincture, as a vapor, capsule and more Accuracy of dosing Full-spectrum Interactions with the full endocannabinoid system, possibly boosting impacts (Ento)

THC WORKING PRINCIPLE

THC is one in all the numerous compounds discovered within the organic compound secreted by the marijuana plant cells. More of these cells are found around the reproductive organs of the plant than in any other region of the plant. Other compounds that are peculiar to marijuana, called cannabinoids, are active in this resin. One cannabinoid, CBD, according to the National Center for Biotechnology Information, is non-psychoactive and effectively prevents the elevated levels connected with THC.

Effects

On the body THC stimulates the brain cells to produce dopamine, generating euphoria according to NIDA. It also interferes with how data is handled in the hippocampus, which is a component of the brain accountable for creating fresh memories.

THC can induce hallucinations, altered thinking, and trigger illusions. On average, the impacts last about two hours and kick in about 10 to 30 minutes after ingestion. Psychomotor impairment may, however, remain after the perceived high has ceased.

"In some instances, recorded side effects of THC include elation, depression, tachycardia, short-term memory problems, sedation, relief, pain relief, and many more," said A.J. Fabrizio, a marijuana chemistry specialist at Terra Tech Corp, a California agricultural business centered on local agriculture and medical cannabis. However, research in the British Journal of Pharmacology discovered that other kinds of cannabinoids, as well as terpenes (compounds that generate flavor and fragrance in crops), can modulate and decrease adverse impacts.

Risks

The impacts of marijuana make it a prevalent drug. In reality, it is regarded to be one of the most widely used illicit drugs in the globe. However, these impacts also affect mental health proponents. According to NIDA, THC can cause a relapse in schizophrenic diseases.

Another feasible danger of THC consumption is in the form of impaired motor skills. Marijuana may impair riding or comparable duties for roughly three hours after eating and is the second most prevalent psychoactive substance discovered in cyclists after alcohol, claims the National Highway Safety Administration. People who take medical marijuana are advised not to ride until it has been identified that they can tolerate it and perform engine duties effectively.

Marijuana use can trigger issues for older individuals and long-term problems. "Some of the side effects of THC include a reduction in IQ, memory, and awareness, particularly among older individuals," said Dr. Damon Raskin, Medical Director at Cliffside Malibu Treatment Centre. "However, the jury is still out on long-term impacts, as not enough research has yet been conducted on it. There is some conjecture that it could impair fertility in males and females, as well as compromise the airways of a person, but the findings are still not evident." A study by the University of Montreal released in Development and Psychopathology in 2016 discovered that early use of marijuana could af if Smokers starting around 14 years of the era do worse than non-smokers on some cognitive tests. A study of nearly 300 students found that pot smokers also had a higher drop-out rate at school. Those who waited to begin around the era of 17 did not seem to have the same impairments.

NIDA states that rats subjected to THC before birth, shortly after birth or during adolescence have had issues with particular teaching and memory functions later in adulthood.

The drug may also have drug relationships with certain medications.

Medical Uses

According to the National Cancer Institute, medicinal uses Marijuana has been used for medicinal purposes for more than 3,000 years. By the end of 2017, more than half of the United States legalized the use of medicinal marijuana. Several nations have also legalized the use of recreation medicines.

THC can be obtained or synthesized from marijuana, as is the situation with the FDA-approved drug dronabinol. Dronabinol is used to cure or discourage nausea and vomiting caused by cancer medications and to boost the appetites of individuals with AIDS, according to the U.S. The National Medical Library. it is a lightweight yellow tarry oil.

CBD'S WORKING PRINCIPLE

The CBD, that was negotiated beneath the auspices of the world organization setting Program (UNEP), was opened for signature at the planet Summit in Rio {de Janeiro Rio city metropolis urban center} de Janeiro on June 1992 and entered into force on twenty-nine Dec 1993. With 191 Parties, the CBD may be a wrongfully binding tool geared toward promoting' the conservation of biological diversity, the property use of its components and therefore the cheap and equitable sharing of benefits ensuing from the utilization of genetic assets.' A landmark in law, the CBD creates the idea of national sovereignty over natural resources. It acknowledges for the first moment that the conservation of biological diversity may be a common issue of grouping and a vital facet of the mechanism of growth. It includes all habitats, species and genetic assets and also addresses the field of biotechnology, including technology transfer and extension, benefit-sharing and biosecurity. It lays out strategies and overall commitments and facilitates technical and economic collaboration. Implementation is, however, needed at the domestic level and the obligation lies with local authorities.

Potential Treatments For Common Ailments

When CBD first hit the market, much of the general public saw it as yet another passing health fad that wouldn't last, however, as more and more research shows that this cannabinoid has the potential to treat a wide range of common diseases, it is clear. That there's something that makes CBD unique. Now, the medical industry is taking note, finding ways to integrate this compound into more conventional treatment methods.

CBD studies show that this plant-based compound can help with everything from digestive disorders to panic attacks. These studies are crucial as they give the public confidence that what they 're taking might help them find relief. And, these studies allow the industry to thrive as it's becoming more and more acceptable to take CBD as an alternative to a more conventional treatment method.

Natural Wellness Boom

Over the last decade, the market for natural health and wellness has become more popular than ever, with more and more people taking an interest in treating their illnesses using natural methods. So, what caused the sudden increase in people who were interested in taking their health into their own hands? Well, part of this has to do with the rise in deaths caused by the misuse of prescription drugs that have become more accessible than ever before.

The opioid crisis has been well documented over the last few years, as statistics show that more people are prescribed popular drugs like Vicodin than ever before. These drugs can be safe if they are taken correctly, but they rarely do. The risk of overdose and dependence on this class of drugs is very high, and as a result, many people have become suspicious of the medical industry for prescribing these drugs so quickly.

The Basics Of CBD

CBD has arrived just as the market for natural health and wellness has been at an all-time high. CBD became accessible to the general public when cannabis laws were amended to classify hemp as a separate substance from marijuana. Suddenly, people could buy hemp-derived CBD products in stores across the country.

According to federal legislation, the CBD sold in stores must come from a hemp plant and must contain no more than 0.3 percent THC, a psychoactive compound that is abundant in marijuana. Because of the low THC content, CBD products that come from hemp won't get you high.

When we speak about CBD, we talk about a bunch about the hemp extract. Hemp is naturally high in CBD, but it also contains other plant compounds which are beneficial. Thus, the majority of CBD products on the market contain CBD in addition to other compounds such as cannabinoids and terpenes that have the potential to provide medicinal benefits.

Why Cbd Becomes A Popular Natural Treatment Option

CBD is becoming more popular every month simply because a lot of people have found it works for them. One thing that makes CBD as potentially useful as an alternative treatment is that it works directly with the endocannabinoid system of the body. Our bodies are producing cannabinoids that the endocannabinoid system sends to the cannabinoid receptors that exist throughout the body. This process allows these body systems to be regulated, which promotes homeostasis.

Researchers now believe that the vast majority of the population is deficient in cannabinoids. It seems, however, that CBD may be able to correct this deficiency. CBD derived from hemp acts as a phytocannabinoid, which means that once it is consumed, the body uses it in the same way that it uses the cannabinoid that it produces itself.

These explain why CBD has the potential to help with such a wide range of illnesses. If cannabinoid receptors exist throughout the body, the endocannabinoid system may send phytocannabinoids to parts of the body that need the most help.

Another advantage that CBD has over popular drugs is that, from now on, it generally seems safe to take daily and in large doses. CBD is non-toxic, which means that there is no risk of a fatal overdose as far as researchers have been able to determine. As a result, many people feel safer taking this compound over popular medicines.

Popular CBD Medicinal Treatments

Due to the popularity of CBD and the recent change in legal status, researchers are finally able to raise funding to study this compound and its potential benefits. Below, you'll discover some of the most popular uses for CBD.

The Potential Of Seizures

CBD to treat epilepsy is very promising. Many researchers have tested their effects on those suffering from seizures with exciting results. CBD appears to have neuroprotective properties as well as a variety of benefits to the neurological system. Since epilepsy is a neurological condition, CBD may be helpful. The FDA recently approved a CBD-based drug for the treatment of epilepsy.

Migraines

More and more migraine sufferers choose to treat their condition with CBD rather than with standard pain medications. Studies show that CBD may be beneficial when it comes to treating this type of headache. It appears that the body's endocannabinoid system controls pain tolerance, which means that the compound can act as a potent analgesic agent.

Arthritis

The treatment of arthritis is another widespread use for CBD. This inflammatory condition affects a large number of people, and the pain may be crippling. CBD may be able to dramatically reduce the inflammation that is responsible for the pain due to its potential ability to control the inflammatory response of the body.

Anxiety

There are many anti-anxiety drugs on the market today, and many of them are addictive. These are partly why so many anxieties sufferers turn to CBD. This cannabinoid may be able to calm the nervous system because of its unique ability to control the amount of cortisol that the brain secretes during moments of stress.

Digestive Upset

Research also shows that CBD may be able to calm the digestive tract, potentially giving it the ability to help with a wide range of gastrointestinal disorders.

High Blood Pressure

Studies have shown that taking CBD daily can help a person manage his or her blood pressure. It seems that a single dose of cannabinoid can reduce blood pressure to a healthy range. This is most likely due to the vital role of endocannabinoid in the regulation of the cardiovascular system.

How CBD Is Taken

CBD is done in several different ways. People can choose between oral tinctures, capsules, edibles, vapor oils, and more. The most important thing is not the type of product you want, but whether or not you take the right dosage level. CBD should be taken daily for the best results, and your dose level depends on your size and the severity of your condition.

It is also essential that you choose a high-quality CBD product because there are many low-quality products on the market today. The higher the quality, the more efficient it can be.

CBD is having success so far CBD is becoming an incredibly popular alternative to conventional treatments because it has the potential to help with different conditions without being as risky as certain drugs. If you would like to treat a disease with CBD, talk to your doctor first.

DOSING CONSIDERATION AND EFFECTS

Dosage of CBD

The ideal amount for the customer relies on several variables, such as body form, CBD tolerance, and the amount of pain or annoyance of the customer. The sort and concentration of the CBD item are other significant factors, as some products communicate differently with the body than others.

This manual will look at all the main factors that need to be taken when determining the correct dosage. We will also show how to assess dosage for distinct CBD products and address some prospective health issues for individuals who eat large quantities of CBD.

Side Effects

Diarrhea Appetite and weight changes CBD fatigue is also considered to communicate with several drugs. Talk to your doctor before you begin using CBD oil to guarantee your safety and prevent possibly damaging relationships.

This is particularly crucial if you are taking medicines or supplements that come with a Grapefruit Warning Grapefruit and CBD interfere with cytochromes P450 (CYP), a class of enzymes that are essential to drug metabolism.

Research on mice has shown that CBD-rich cannabis extracts are capable of causing hepatic toxicity. However, some of the mice in the study were injected with massive amounts of the extract.

Although CBD is usually deemed secure, some individuals may experience negative responses such as diarrhea and fatigue. It may also interfere with certain medicines.

HOW TO BUY SAFE, QUALITY PRODUCTS

CBD in the globe of wellness right now? The market is exploding with what is affectionately referred to as the "green boom," with everything from CBD bath bombs Protein powder and CBD lube marketed at every corner of the Internet. You don't need to discover a local dispensary-because CBD is legal everywhere, and you can purchase it online with very few constraints.

When Buying Cbd Gets Scary

But beware: while there are loads of incredible cannabis-based health and wellness products out there for buy, CBD is still brand new and therefore unregulated. Just like dietary supplements, the FDA does not strictly monitor the development and delivery of CBD-so products are not under strict scrutiny when it relates to how they concoct, label, and distribute their cannabis products.

"There is a lot of excellent development going on right now, but because it's a fresh sector, there are also fly-by-night competitors looking to create a fast buck," said Joel Stanley, chairman and one of the developers of Charlotte's Web CBD oil. "In reality, the FDA carried out its survey of CBD products and discovered that many do not even contain CBD," he said. "Knowing what is in products is a major purchase concern for new CBD consumers, and we believe that regulation and consumer education are so important right now." The study, published in the Journal of the American Medical Association in November 2017, found that about 26% of the CBD products tested contained a significant amount of CBD products tested. Less CBD per milliliter than the label advertised.

NBC New York also chose to evaluate commercially available CBD products, and the findings did not look great. Their investigative group screened three products of CBD oil and four types of gums, buying five samples of each brand. They tested them in a third-party laboratory and discovered that less than half of the samples collected effectively had the specified quantity of CBD inside the item, that one brand had no CBD whatsoever in its product, that one brand had a pesticide that exceeded the appropriate California norms, and, shockingly, that another had four times the quantity of lead!) (permitted by the FDA.

Because this whole space is so new, most people don't even understand that there are some red flags or stuff to look for when shopping for a secure, high-quality, sheer CBD item. How do you ensure that what you put on or put in your body is, in fact, legal or even safe?

First things, don't fear. Here, some of the most reliable funds in the cannabis sector give their knowledge on how to purchase CBD safely-because, without regulation in place, you have to "regulate" yourself. Here's what you need to look for, what you need to prevent, and everything you need to understand while shopping for CBD.

Buy from the Right Brands Getting to understand the brand legitimately counts in cannabis room. Fortunately, many businesses are doing their role by being transparent and offering customers the information they need.

"The main differentiator when it goes to purchasing a secure and reliable CBD] is getting to know the brand," said Kiana Reeves, CEO of Foria Wellness (which produces some beautiful cannabis products for sexual health). "When you begin researching any marijuana, CBD, or wellness business, look at how much they learn, how much data they're giving out not just transparency and components, but forward-thinking practices." "Look for a brand that's not just placing random isolates into a cosmetic item, but researching what's most useful to the client and demonstrating where they're going to get. "The more confidence and efficacy you can build, the superior you will be." Stanley reflected this concept, instructing CBD customers to look at the brand and their capacity to regulate what they call the "farm-to-shelf" process. Florida is one of those companies–as Reeves has informed us, Foria employees have "profoundly private interactions with growers and producers," which enables them to be more in touch with the intricacy of their manufacturing.

Get the Certificate of Analysis (COA) "Without a lab report, the tag can mean anything," tells chiropractor Allen Miller, D.C., Director of Operations at Doctors Cannabis Consulting and Calm Consultant at Wellness Co. When it goes to confidence, as Reeves said, you're only going to want to purchase from a business that offers a COA, or an evaluation certificate. This small PDF is proof that a third-party, independent laboratory has tested the product you are about to purchase and found several things, including the following super-important ones.

Something to maintain in mind: you're going to want to understand the batch amount of the CBD item you're looking at, tells Megan Villa, co-founder of the Hemp-focused blog and Shop Space. "Ask the COA for the batch amount of the item you have, as these products are produced in batches," she said. "You need to match the batch amount to the COA that belongs to it." Potency: Is there a CBD in there? How much is that? Look for "complete cannabinoids" or "complete CBD" in the COA. "Potency informs you the number of cannabinoids in the item," Villa said. "If a brand and product claim 250 mg of CBD, this should be consistent with what is stated in the COA." (Shared a reference COA that ticks all the correct boxes.)

Contaminants or pesticides: was hemp cultivated in pesticide-soaked soil? Did this get into the item? Was the CBD extracted with solvents? Are they in the subject, huh? "Request batch screening results to ensure there are no contaminants, toxins, heavy metals, etc.," suggests Stanley. "Each business should not only carry out in-house tests but also check through reliable third-party laboratories that the item has the right concentration of CBD and is safe of contaminants, remaining solvents, and pesticides."

"This guarantees that there is no mold or bacteria in the hemp used to create your CBD item." Safety: while hundreds of new CBD businesses are flowing up every day, pharmacist Earl Mindell, Ph.D., at Calm by Wellness Co., invites customers to "discover a company that has been in business for more than three years." Mindell observed that it would be simpler for them to demonstrate that the laboratories they use are in business for more than three years.

Buy Domestic Sourced Hemp

"You want to understand the source of the hemp used in your item," Stanley said. "Hemp is a strong phytoremediation plant, which implies that it cleans the soil." (It is also referred to as a bioaccumulator.) This implies that when hemp is grown, it absorbs everything that is in the soil around it, including toxins, heavy metals, pesticides, and nuclear fallout. You'll want to guarantee that the hemp in your item is cultivated using accountable soil farming methods that are pre-tested for toxins, suggests Stanley. Reeves also emphasized this, stating that how hemp is grown is equivalent to its safety as a consumer product.

"Look for CBD products produced from American-grown hemp (including New York, Colorado, Kentucky, Oregon, Vermont, Tennessee, etc.)," tells Melany Dobson, Chief Administrative Officer of Hudson Hemp, because they are usually safer than foreign-grown hemp.

"California has one of the best products in the globe coming out of the' green triangle' in Humboldt County," tells Miller. Ben Odell at Foria Wellness also pointed to the California industry, referencing Flow Kana, a California-based sustainable cannabis farming cooperative that brought together craft growers.

Aim For CO2-Extract Products

"Concerning searching at the pesticide lab records, how it was cultivated and the level of metal, you'll want to learn more about how it was produced," tells Miller. "I am a supporter of CO2 extraction because it is non-toxic." Alternatives are butane or ethanol-based extraction. Both chemicals can end up in your item. You're supposed to be prepared to see that in the COA.

Reading The Label

Label for CBD is an sh*t show right now because there's so much government gray area (and the FDA isn't helping out). But, according to Odell, if the item mentions "CBD" on it, it could even be a red flag. "Technically, the FDA could come down on you to print' CBD' on your item," states Odell. "Charlotte's Web is an example of this; they are the largest, most reputable brand, and indeed the founders in space, and they no longer print' CBD' on their stuff." Many products now say "hemp extract" due to pressure from the FDA and DEA-because, according to them, if a product is listed as a dietary supplement, it can not contain CBD (see the above remark about the FDA not being a nutritional additive). It may tell "hemp extract" with specified cannabidiol milligrams, but most products have exchanged labels to be secure.

Plus, printing "CBD" is not very revealing. "If it just says CBD, is it insulation? An extract? You don't understand.

Consider Full-or Broad-Spectrum Hemp Instead of CBD Isolate,' Ask if the item is full-spectrum,' suggests Stanley. "Hemp has many useful compounds beyond CBD, and all of these compounds operate together, constructing on their strengths to further enhance the body's favorable reaction to CBD." "Isolate is extremely inexpensive and not as efficient; broad-spectrum is balanced," adds Odell, who defines the "U-shaped dose-response curve" when it goes to CBD isolation, stating, "As the dosage rises, its effect is balanced." "You're not supposed to murder yourself by having an insulator, but you want a full-plant, broad-spectrum item And even if it's CBD insulator, it can still be more efficient than aspirin," Dobson said. "Both pure CBD and full-spectrum CBD with its phytocannabinoids were more efficient than aspirin in alleviating both inflammation and pain," Broad-Spectrum vs.

In contrast, the broad-spectrum is distilled and removes certain compounds, leaving the sample with' a total proportion of a single cannabinoid (most frequently CBD) with a broad spectrum of associated cannabinoids and terpenes,' Caution: Avoid Hemp Seed Oil Hemp Seed Oil does not match CBD:' CBD is not obtained from the seed and stem of the hemp plant because[the compound] is not the same as CBD.

Odell and Reeves also advised that hemp seed oil sold in big-box internet shops like Amazon would be marketed as CBD. You're receiving something nearer to olive oil than real medicine. (Just a heads up: you can't purchase CBD on Amazon. "If you're looking for a CBD product on Amazon, you'll see a lot of stuff that's hemp seed oil—they're attempting to catch unwitting individuals," said Odell. " Hemp seed oil is good; it's full of omega-3s, nutritious and all that, but there's very little (if any) CBD." Know Your Resources Each company you buy from should have a help squad to address the question.

AN OVERVIEW OF THE ENDOCANNABINOID SYSTEM

Have you ever noticed how cannabinoids interact with your body? The endocannabinoid system is the answer.

The endocannabinoid system is responsible for regulating the balance of our body's immune response, appetite, metabolism, memory, and more. Despite the vital role that this system performs, it remained an unknown element of the human body's duties until recently.

Named for the plant that led to its growth, the importance of the endocannabinoid system is being understood only by the medical society. It is through this scheme that natural cannabinoids from medical cannabis communicate with our organs and cause their positive impacts. With the ability to have a significant effect on the manner our body works, it is vital that we acknowledge how to keep a sound endocannabinoid system.

What's the Endocannabinoid System?

The endocannabinoid system consists of several embedded mechanisms: enzymes accountable for the creation and destruction of cannabinoid receptor locations on cannabinoid-receiving neurons (CB1 and CB2) of endocannabinoids themselves (compounds generated by the human body).

Together, these mechanisms are primarily accountable for controlling the procedures and functions of the body.

Endocannabinoids communicate with CB1 and CB2 receptor locations to help the body attain homeostasis or balance2.

The CB1 and CB2 receptors react differently to distinct cannabinoids, respectively. CB1 receptors, most common in the central nervous system, are associated with modulating pressure, fear, hunger, nausea, immune system equilibrium, and even tumor inhibition1. CB2 receptors, most commonly discovered on cells in the immune system, appear to dominate inflammation control and tissue damage. Some batteries may also comprise both kinds of receptors, each accountable for a distinct feature.

Phytocannabinoids, which are compounds discovered in cannabis seeds, stalks, and flowers, also communicate with cannabinoid receptors. The most prevalent cannabinoids found in cannabis are tetrahydrocannabinol (THC), a psychoactive compound known to generate elevated levels, and cannabidiol (CBD), a non-psychoactive compound.

While the endocannabinoid system is connected to a variety of significant mechanisms and is focused on the brain, nervous system, and reproductive organs, it has not been shown to influence areas of the brain that regulate heart and lung function. This is one of the primary factors that there is no deadly overdose of cannabinoids.

How To Stimulate The Endocannabinoid System Without Cannabis

When individuals learn about all the different health circumstances that cannabis can assist with, some might ask how one herb can have so many strong medical characteristics without any severe side effects.

This issue resulted in scientists to find a physiology scheme that works within all of us to continuously preserve homeostasis or equilibrium at the cellular stage. The endogenous cannabinoid model (endocannabinoid) was named after the plant that resulted in its discovery. It is one of the most important physiological processes engaged in the development and maintenance of human health.

Most of us don't understand that our bodies have been producing cannabinoids all the time. These molecules are very similar to THC and the other cannabinoids discovered in the plant. Our cells generate and use cannabinoids precisely to react to stress, disease, and accident, maintaining you safe. Evidence exists that some people's endocannabinoid system (ECS) may not function optimally; this can be resolved by introducing the correct dosage of additional cannabis cannabinoids.

Beyond cannabis, however, certain products and operations can also assist the ECS to work optimally, improve your health, and improve the efficacy of medical marijuana.

Endocannabinoid-Enhancing Foods Essential fatty acids, cocoa, herbs, spices, and tea may naturally enhance ECS

Essential carboxylic acid a decent proportion of omega-3 fatty acid and polyunsaturated fatty acid fatty acids might improve ECS activity. Endocannabinoids area unit manufactured from polyunsaturated fatty acid carboxylic acid arachidonic acid. Having enough arachidonic acid is significant for the manufacture of endocannabinoids, however obtaining an excessive amount of will contribute to a discount within the regulation of cannabinoid receptors. (Excessive polyunsaturated fatty acid consumption is additionally pro-inflammatory. Most Western diets already involve surplus polyunsaturated fatty acid oils, usually found in preparation oils like herb, sunflower, maize and soybean, and in animal merchandise like pork, chicken, and eggs.) omega-3 fatty acid fatty acids area unit needed to balance polyunsaturated fatty acid fats so the ECS will perform adequately. These fatty acids area unit way tougher to develop in diet and have additionally been shown to possess vas and neurologic health edges. The best proportion of omega-3 fatty acid to polyunsaturated fatty acid within the food is usually typical for western foods. Animal sources of omega-3 fat acid area unit the foremost powerful, however, feeder sources tend to supply alternative necessary health edges.

Sources of endocannabinoid-enhancing fatty acids: hemp seeds and hemp petroleum Flax seeds (measuring reception in tiny mollusks) and oil Chia Walnuts Sardinia and anchovies Eggs (pasture-fed or omega-3-enriched only) 5 Things Chemically Similar to Cannabis High Chocolate Cacao powder includes three compounds that are structurally very comparable to endocannabinoids.

These compounds may prevent the decomposition of your body's endocannabinoids, leading in higher concentrations of endocannabinoid, and may have some cannabinoid activity of their own. The level of cannabinoid-like compounds in chocolate differs extensively and is most significant in dark chocolate and coarse cocoa. Other chocolate compounds may assist avoid heart disease, stroke, and dementia. Look for at least 70% dark chocolate, or try adding raw cocoa nibs to smoothies or cereal!

Herbs And Tea

Numerous herbs and teas contain compounds that may improve ECS. Beta-caryophyllene is a terpene discovered in black pepper, citrus balm, hops, cloves, cannabis, oregano, cinnamon, and several other herbs. It selectively stimulates the CB2 receptor, a sought-after feature in the growth of medicines for inflammatory illnesses.

Echinacea, often used by herbalists for up to two decades to boost the immune system during infection, also includes CB2 agonists.

Camelia Sinensis, frequently referred to as tea, includes a compound that avoids the breakdown of endocannabinoids and another synthesis that may boost the receptors of cannabinoids.

Turmeric, a yellow spice in curry powder, contains curcumin, which also increases endocannabinoid levels among many other health benefits.

Certain pesticides (e.g., chlorpyrifos and piperonyl butoxide) are considered to interfere with ECS. It is particularly essential to choose organic food when shopping for food, milk, and the most significant pesticide-containing products. Phthalates, commonly added to plastic and tin metal containers and cans of water, are considered to block cannabinoid receptors and interrupt the body's hormonal system. Choose glass or stainless steel food containers and packaging whenever possible and never eat food that is heated in plastic.

Alcohol

Regular use of mild to elevated amounts of alcohol may also impair ECS, so for ideal safety and endocannabinoid function, use moderation when smoking or prevent drinking in its entirety.

Endocannabinoid-Enhancing Activities

Certain operations can enhance the functioning of the ECS, improve your health, boost the efficacy of medicinal cannabis, and assist you to feel good.

Stress-Reducing Activities

While chronic stress can deplete your ECS, a strongly customized ECS can safeguard you from the harmful impacts of tension. Incorporating practice into your routine will hold your ECS tuned, but only if you appreciate it! Animal studies tell us that if you allow yourself to practice, your ECS will perceive the activity as stress, but selecting and loving the same event can have the reverse impact of stress and boost the level of endocannabinoids. Socializing can also be useful for reducing stress and improving the ECS function. In social isolation, rats generated fewer cannabinoid receptors, while social play and grooming conduct improved ECS activity.

Here are a few proposed endocannabinoid-enhancing and health-enhancing activities: social interaction Unstructured playtime (this is essential for adolescents too!) Meditation Yoga Massage Osteopathic Manipulation (OMT) Acupuncture Breathing sessions Voluntary and fun exercise The wellness segment at Healer.com offers simple activities that are easy for everyone and pleasant.

Endocannabinoids and their receptors are detected throughout the body: in the brain, organs, connective tissue, glands, and immune cells. The cannabinoid mechanism conducts distinct duties in each fabric, but the objective is always the same: homeostasis, the preservation of a stable inner setting despite changes in the external environment. Your body generates cannabinoids of its own. Proper cannabis dosages can also up-regulate and tone your ECS. However, the plant is not the only way to promote your ECS. You can boost your ECS with delicious endocannabinoid-enhancing ingredients and pleasant operations that can contribute to significant health advantages.

The History Of The Endocannabinoid System

Throughout the 19th century, cannabis plant extracts have been widely used for several medicinal purposes in the United States.

Fearing the abuse of Cannabis ' psychoactive properties, the federal government forbade the cannabis plant in 1937. This prevented the plant from being used for recreation, medicine, and research, which ended up stalling the progress of our understanding of the endocannabinoid system and the potential therapeutic properties. For almost 50 years, cannabis has been removed from popular pharmacopeia and labeled illegal in the minds of most Americans.

However, in the mid-1990s, Lisa Matsuda and her crew at the National Institute of Mental Health first recognized a THC-sensitive receptor in rat brains. After this revelation, the National Academy of Sciences predicted that the 1990s would be the "Decade of the Brain." It turned out to be true that the next 10-year period would bring "more advances in neuroscience than all previous years combined"5.

Since then, researchers have been collaborating to know as much as they can about the endocannabinoid system, our naturally occurring cannabinoids, and how cannabis alters this equilibrium, releasing over 20,000 cannabinoid-referencing science papers over the last two centuries.

How Does The Endocannabinoid System Influence My Health?

Since the development of the endocannabinoid system and its elements, the scientists have struggled to know further how the endocannabinoid system can be used therapeutically to decrease pain, combat cancer, deter neurodegenerative diseases and encourage wellness. Overall, the study demonstrates that the endocannabinoid system helps to control the body's immune and central nervous processes and guarantees that they function correctly.

One hypothesis on how the endocannabinoid system contributes to our general wellness is the endocannabinoid deficiency syndrome, which speculates that the body does not generate enough endocannabinoids for some people. This idea further thinks that weakness can be the root cause of many autoimmune disorders, including migraine, fibromyalgia, irritable bowel syndrome, and more.

Overall, the critical study is still needed to comprehend better the effect of the endocannabinoid system on our general health and how supplementing our natural endocannabinoid manufacturing with plant-based cannabinoids can play an essential beneficial function in our health.

THE DIFFERENCE BETWEEN INDICA, SATIVA, AND HYBRIDS

You've probably heard these words before, but do you understand what they imply? Cannabis is classified into two species: Indica and Sativa (don't worry, there's a point in this precise class). In addition to the two, you can also have "blends" of the two in different proportions called Hybrids.

There are many variations between the anatomy of the two animals: how they are cultivated, how long they take to flower, and more, but one of the most significant distinctions is the chemicals they generate, and what that implies for the customers of these products. Below is a more comprehensive description of the three which should shed light on it. Is it still mistaken? You can discover more info here when we get to know more about the distinct times for cannabis use.

Keep in mind that the potential impacts below do not necessarily extend to all individuals. Your distinctive biology, expectations, and background of cannabis will dictate how you respond concerning your environments and environments.

India

Most Known for getting a physical sedative effect on the body Often selected for: quiet times, pre-sleep consumption, low-impact activities at home Looks like: brief, stocky crops with broad leaves Origin: India (although the evolving study has suggested that it may merely originate in Afghanistan)

Sativa

Most Known for mental effects Often selected for: physical exercise, sociology Hybrids can be either Indica or Sativa dominant in their genetic structure and impact. Each element could contribute something distinct to the overall experience. Strains can be developed to allow the different characteristics of the two relatives to merge and to generate something different from either of the two plants on their own.

Other Active Cannabis

Cannabis also recognized as marijuana, weed, pot, or a thousand other names this drug appears to have maybe extremely addictive to some individuals who are struggling to stop smoking cannabis. In this scenario, how to stop smoking cannabis depends on knowing marijuana and its impacts on your mind and body. Only then will you be prepared to feel the advantages of quitting smoking cannabis and be ready to remain away from weed and not relapse into your addiction.

First of all, we need to realize that there are some misconceptions about cannabis addiction that contribute to individuals attempting to remove pot-smoking incorrectly and can also provide to pro-marijuana consumers ridicule the concept of addiction that is unhelpful to everyone concerned.

Cannabis is not physically addictive Many surveys have shown that smoking marijuana is not like smoking cigarettes, where the chemicals (nicotine) render you physically addicted to drugs, and when hungry, you die from cravings that cause you to burn again to be free of the consequences. This does not imply that preventing cannabis smoking does not come with a collection of desires, but they are usually of a distinct kind.

Cannabis Withdrawals

Cannabis withdrawals are prevalent when you give up smoking weeds, but any physical cravings are very gentle but can include: Vividdreams-I'm not sure what triggers them, but many individuals coming out of cannabis often discover their memories very vivid and sometimes frightening. This may have something to do with the chemical THC that remains in your body for decades after you quit using it.

Anxiety-The feeling of paranoia and stress can be heightened while you're working on the chemicals out of your body.

Insomnia-Some individuals have indicated that it is hard to sleep, which may again be linked to your body's readjustment.

These symptoms go on in the moment and are generally nothing like the horrible consequences of quitting cigarettes, and the actual cravings originate from your psychological dependence on the drug that has to do with your wishing it not to be physically needed!

Psychological Dependence

Psychological dependence is when you think you need to smoke cannabis in the form of joints, bongs, or whatever you choose as you believe you need it. This is complicated, and sometimes you may not understand why you feel that you have to smoke, but for most individuals, it is because it has become a practice to burn to flee from something in your own lives. From fleeing violence, poverty, mental illness, depression or just being tired and unmotivated, you can be the victim of smoking weed because you need to escape from your truth and the high you get is a short-term comfort that keeps things bearable for a while. This is not a long-term option, though, and ongoing smoking often makes it worse and solves nothing that leads to a spiraling pit of depression, frustration, and even more cannabis dependence to get through it all.

So how to avoid smoking cannabis? The first stage is to understand what you've just read and found out when you choose to use marijuana. Only from there can you expect to take action to prevent the drug and achieve the advantages of better thinking, more time in your lives to alter stuff, and more cash to modify things. Make it happen!

If you want to understand how you can make this shift happen, stop smoking cannabis

THE RISKS OF SMOKING MARIJUANA

The impact and risk of smoking marijuana are highest in the adolescent ages. An individual who smokes marijuana will have issues dealing with interpersonal skills. They're going to have trouble knowing stuff because the chemical of marijuana impacts their brains. Cannabis is regularly used as a drug portal. According to studies undertaken at the Center for Addiction and Substance Abuse, adolescents are more probable to smoke weed eighty-five times than cocaine. Research also indicates that 60 percent of young people use cocaine after using marijuana.

Marijuana is going to affect the decision and perception of the individual. When a person gets grass, he will not be prepared to run a machine. As a consequence, he's not going to be fit to ride a vehicle. Driving a vehicle under the impact of marijuana will improve the likelihood of an incident. Many youthful individuals experience car accidents and get severely wounded when riding under the effects of marijuana. Hemp is also a significant source of casual sex and sexually transmitted diseases (STDs). Cannabis may trigger temporary memory loss for at least 24 hours. The person will have a quicker heartbeat frequency and will suffer from anxiety. Society underplays the impacts of smoking marijuana, yet this has such a substantial effect on our daily living marijuana that it will trigger a hormonal imbalance. When a person experiences a hormonal imbalance, the start of puberty is lighter. Males will have poor sperm manufacturing issues. Females are going to have uneven menstrual problems. Pregnant women who smoke pot will offer birth to children who have an issue with their health. The chemicals in marijuana will trigger the child to experience deformation. Premature birth may also occur when a pregnant mom smokes marijuana. Children have an elevated chance of having emotional and physical developmental delays. If you don't want your kid to become a handicap, you're not supposed to smoke weed. Consequently, the impacts of smoking marijuana are disastrous. You should not stop smoking marijuana without considering the effects that can occur to yourself and your child.

Marijuana is often used as a pain relief medication to relieve patients of symptoms such as glaucoma, AIDS, and cancer. However, the study has not shown that marijuana can reduce side effects better than authorized medicine. You should make up your mind to stop smoking after you realize the impacts of smoking marijuana. Making your account stop smoking right now can save your lives and prevent further problems. If you think that you lack motivation, you can always seek support from your colleagues. You're supposed to get rid of all the marijuana, so you don't have access to it. You're not going to fall into relapse in this manner.

Your Body On Marijuana

When you consume pot, THC and other chemicals move from the bloodstream to your brain. THC creates the feeling-good' high.' Here are some of the other impacts you'll feel:

- Trouble thinking and remembering
- Bloodshot eyes
- Dry mouth (cottonmouth)
- Increased appetite(' munchies')
- Fast heart rate
- Slowed coordination

Marijuana Smoke: What's In It?

Marijuana smoke contains approximately 60 chemicals called cannabinoids. The best known of these is THC, which also contributes to the indications that someone was smoking pot: memory loss and random ideas, as well as a steadfast stroll.

Marijuana includes many of the same chemicals discovered in cigarette smoke and many in larger quantities. Tar, for instance, is more focused in marijuana smoke than in cigarette smoke.

Smoking marijuana leads the heart to run and the mouth to dry and the eyes to get bloodshot.

Studies indicate that the drug can harm your short-term memory, warp your natural feeling of the moment, change your perception of depth by slowing down your reflexes, and slowing down your reaction time.

Marijuana smoke includes 50 to 70 percent more of cancer that causes the chemicals that smoke the cigarette. Marijuana smoke generates elevated concentrations of an enzyme that alters certain hydrocarbons in their carcinogenic shape and may further boost the danger of carcinogenic structures.

Research shows that THC, a psychoactive component in marijuana, impairs the capacity of the immune systems to combat diseases, cancer cells, and shapes.

Smoking marijuana at all raises the danger of chronic cough, bronchitis, and emphysema, but frequent smoking leads to a more significant risk factor.

Personality changes and emotional problems have been favorably related to the use of marijuana. Depression, hopelessness, and other psychological issues are often aggravated by smoking weeds. This involves the intensification of pre-existing mental disturbances.

Studies have shown that early use of marijuana improves the probability of other, often more addictive and possibly life-threatening drugs being abused.

For some individuals, marijuana use contributes to addiction, including compulsive drug-seeking, physical, emotional and mental withdrawal signs, and ongoing drug use despite harmful effects and repeated efforts to prevent it.

While it may seem otherwise, after you've been out of weed for a while, you'll understand that life is more comfortable when you stand on your own, without doing it to have fun or relax.

SAFE WAYS TO CONSUME MEDICAL MARIJUANA

How you handle, it is up to you to eat medical marijuana. In your body, each technique operates differently. Smoking or spraying will create you feel the impacts of cannabis almost immediately. However, it may take up to 2 hours for edibles to become active.

Smoke it Inhale through a machine called a vaporizer that transforms it into a mist Eat it for instance, in a brownie or lollipop Apply it to your body in a lotion, cream, soap or cream Place a few drops of fluid under your tongue. Medical marijuana is a very effective medication used by clients around the world to cure and relieve signs of many severe medical circumstances that do not react. Studies have shown that cannabis has therapeutic properties that can not be replicated by any other presently prescribed medication and that it produces far less and much less severe side effects than many frequently prescribed pharmaceuticals and counter-drugs.

One of the first issues that nurses often ask us is: "What are the finest and healthiest methods to eat medical cannabis?"First, unless you reside in a state like Colorado, Washington or Oregon that allows for recreational marijuana buys and use, and depending on the legislation of your country, you will need a medical marijuana advice letter and medical cannabis card from your doctor. This phase generally involves an in-person interview and testing method so that the doctor can determine if cannabis is a healthy option for you.

First of all, being depersonalized does not imply that you are depressed, nor does it suggest that you become psychotic. Depersonalization is just a demonstration of anxiety, a weak emotion that skews your life perspective, and that's why you want to address the fundamental concern to get rid of the dissociation. Luckily, there are a lot of methods that will allow a full rehabilitation, and these are the ones I discovered most effective: identifying the sources-although anxiety is mostly an irrational sensation due to neuro-biological malfunctions, each of us will have some environmental and chemical causes, such as public speaking, discovering fresh regions, drinking alcohol/coffee, smoking, etc. Each of us will have a distinct number of these irritants, so it's essential to locate them so that you can tackle them correctly. Getting a general idea of what anxiety is, how it presents itself, and its mechanism of intervention can be extremely helpful in managing stress and managing depersonalization as well. Adapting this strategy makes it simpler to differentiate your weight from your true self, which is an essential step towards rehabilitation.

Exposure therapy-Addressing the environmental triggers of your anxiety that you have effectively recognized may sound uncomfortable and may seem counter-productive at first, but the long-term effects are worth the initial fear. What it does to expose yourself to trigger-situations such as being among the masses of individuals is to desensitize your nervous reactions, ultimately enabling you to flourish in an earlier anticipated, aversive scenario. Start low, with the gentle implementation of the trigger(s) if you think it's too much to manage, and if you achieve trust, move it up a lot more again.

Occupying your mind-you might have realized that anxiety takes the most benefit of you when you let your mind roam, bringing unpleasantly intrusive thoughts into your consciousness. An excellent solution to this issue is to spend your concentrate on some exercise, whether it's playing the piano or walking on a hot, sunny day. Activities consume your ideas and concentrate, leaving no room for worrying thoughts, and besides, you do something useful and thus think great about yourself.

Implementing and adhering to the above methods is one of the most effective panaceas in fighting anxiety, the real culprit behind marijuana-induced depersonalization. From my knowledge, the use of prescription drugs continues to hinder the entire recovery cycle, although they may be helpful in urgent cases. These three methods have been an excellent assistance to me in overcoming my depersonalization, and there are many more that could do the trick. In the resource chapter, I have included a connection to a long list of such methods so that you can choose the most attractive to you. Techniques that operated less for me could function better for you, and vice versa, so I promote you to experiment. Now go ahead, get involved, and appreciate going back to your ancient self!

Once you have obtained your proposal and your card, you will be free to enter and purchase different types of cannabis from a local or community marijuana dispensary. Smoking cannabis flowers is a well-known method of administration (or "medicine"), but there are many alternative ways to profit from medicinal cannabis, each with specific benefits and disadvantages.

Smoking Medical Cannabis

How It Works: pack a small amount of dried (cured) cannabis crop into a pipe, a water tube (bong) or a rolling paper (to create a "joint").

Keep the fire on the cannabis flower until it sheds as you inhale the smoke from the mouthpiece or the other side of the joint.

Pros

- Delivers instant relief
- Fairly easy to regulate dosage
- Inexpensive
- Minimally processed
- Multiple options

Smoking may be detrimental to the lungs. Studies have reached contradictory findings as to whether and to what extent cannabis can trigger lung harm, but the burning of any material makes it more difficult to breathe.

In many instances, not a healthy choice for anyone with lung harm (lung cancer, emphysema) or asthma Will make you smell like marijuana smoke Dosage: start low! Lightly inhale (i.e. "take a tiny shot"). There is no need to keep the smoke in your lungs... to exhale. Wait a couple of minutes. If you don't feel the required impact, or if you want to experience a higher result, bring another shot.

Vaporizing" Vaping" Medical Marijuana

How It Works: Preheat the vaporizer at the suggested temperature. Insert a tiny quantity of dried (healed) marijuana flower or extract into a vaporizer. Press the button to inhale. Cannabis is heated to a temperature below its combustion stage, but still warm enough to free the herbal compounds.

Vaporizers are accessible in a broad range of shapes and sizes, from fancy home appliances to pocket-friendly pens.

Pros

- Delivers Instant
- Relief Less severe on the lungs than smoking
- Don't make you smell as much as smoking

Cons

- Vaping Units can be very costly.
- The battery-powered devices must be recharged.
- Need time for the unit to heat up.

Dosage: Start the little one! Lightly inhale (i.e. "take a tiny shot"). There is no need to keep the smoke in your lungs to exhale. Wait a couple of minutes. If you don't feel the required impact, or if you want to experience a higher result, bring another shot.

Medical Marijuana Edibles

How It Operates: once, food was restricted to homemade brownies that tasted fairly horrible and contained a mysterious dose of THC. Nowadays, you can discover medicated cookies, popcorn, crackers, nut mixtures, lollipops, ice cream, gum bears, chocolate bars, chews, and many other foods. Culinary science has developed enough to make most of the products yummy that you can hardly say they contain cannabis.

Pros

- Provides long-term relief.
- Good option for individuals who do not want to inhale.
- You're going to consume a delightful treat.
- The dosage can be very accurate.

Cons

- It can take half an hour or several hours to kick in.
- Dosage can be hard for the maker.
- It has to be shut up to prevent kids and animals.
- It's a distinct "heavy" than smoking.

Most Popular: this is the most common technique among children and elderly patients.

Dosage: Only use edibles under the guidance of a physician. Dosages differ extensively based on your weight, metabolism, amount of knowledge, and other variables. Doctors we understand have proposed beginning with a tiny quantity of 2 mg or less and waiting at least an hour to eat more.

Medical Marijuana Tinctures Or Sub-Lingual Sprays

How It Operates: extracted cannabinoids are combined with alcohol, glycerin solution or MCT Oil (Medium-Chain Triglycerides), which in many instances is coconut oil. Usually, these sublingual products come in a tiny bottle. Just squirt or push it under your tongue and let it flow through the soft tissue of your mouth.

Pros

- Don't harm your lungs like inhaling cannabis.
- Easy to regulate the dose at a minimal dose.
- The mild flavor of it.
- I have preferred child technique.

Cons

- May be costly for individuals who take a hefty dose of cannabinoids.
- Effects quicker than edibles, but not as quickly as inhalation.

Dosage: Start with a few falls and wait 10 minutes. If you don't feel relieved, attempt a few more falls. Eventually, you'll find out your perfect dosage for most individuals, and it's between half a dropper and a few droppers at the moment.

Medical Cannabis Transdermal Patches

How It Operates: Apply the patch to a smooth, smooth, hairless skin layer. Many medical experts suggest that the brace be attached to the inside of the wrist, to the top of the foot or the ankle. This is the perfect technique for any patient who prefers not to inhale the medicine. If you've tried various alternatives without achievement, this might be the correct route to take depending on your big decision you're attempting to achieve.

Pros

- No Smoking Required.
- It comes in distinct formulations.
- Mild dosage.

Cons

- Some people may create allergic reactions.
- It must be added to a smooth and fresh surface of the skin.
- Not to be implemented where there is a lot of body hair.

Dosage: Most transdermal pads are available in 10 mg dosed pads. They can be split in half at lower doses.

Medical Marijuana Suppositories

How it operates: you put a tiny, cone-shaped piece of cannabis paste into the rectum where it is absorbed through the colon. This technique is somewhat contentious and less dignified than any other method of medicine, but some nurses swear by it. Put on the protective gloves, lay down on your side, and place the suppository in about 1.5 inches. Squeeze the tissues of your sphincter and remain in position for at least a few minutes. When you're prepared, get up, toss back your gloves, and wash your hands carefully. There are also firms that create pre-made proportions of rectal medicines– 1 mg non-injectable syringes.

Pros

- An excellent option for food.
- Kicks in a fast and long manner to digest the most efficient way.

Cons

- Painful and awkward to manage.
- It has to be refrigerated.
- It's difficult to apply.

Dosage: Most of the suppositories come in two sizes: 2 g for adults and 1 g for kids. They can be split in half at lower doses.

Medical Marijuana Topicals

How It Operates: Medical cannabis tinctures are an excellent way to medicate without psychoactive effects. Salves, ointments, lotions, and sprays are good for arthritis, chapped skin, eczema, minor wounds, muscle aches, sunburns, swelling, joint pain, and tendonitis, to mention but a few.

Pros

- Topicals don't get you "high."
- Addressing skin problems
- Localized pain relief

Cons

- Does not assist cancer, PTSD, epilepsy, or glaucoma.
- Don't give a sensation of euphoria.
- Patients report that some products don't function.

Dosage: You are unlikely to cause any actual damage to the topicals, but attempt to discover those that are targeted to your particular illness. Use salves and ointments as often as you want, keeping in mind that they can get sticky. If you have a skin rash, stop using it. Consult your doctor about the use of transdermal patches.

Ingesting Fresh Medical Cannabis

How it operates: Raw cannabis has evolved quite a bit. Patients argue that the raw plant has medicinal properties that are wasted when the plant is washed or heated. You ingest the fresh leaves and seeds directly from the plant, generally by blending them in a juice or a smoothie.

Pros

- Raw cannabis is filled with THC-A, an acidic type of THC that is not psychoactive. Some patients and physicians think that THC-A has distinctive medicinal properties.
- Some people whose chronic diseases have never replied to other treatments (including frozen cannabis) claim that juicing raw marijuana has been a miracle cure.

Cons

- Requires a significant amount of new cannabis.
- It has an unpleasant flavor for vegetables.
- The findings of studies have not been verified.

Dosage: Dr. William Courtney, a significant proponent of juicing, proposes a weekly intake of 15 leaves and one or two large flowers

Medical Marijuana Beverages

How It Operates: Your local dispensary is likely to sell cans of cannabis teas, juices, smoothies and sodas. You can also create your cannabis tea by steeping a flower, glue, or tincture in warm water. Adding a bag of your favorite beverage can enhance your taste.

Pros

- Provides long-term relief.
- Alternative for individuals who do not want to inhale their medicine.
- Give a particular sensation, such as stress relief or energy.

Cons

- Takes about 30min-2hours to kick in.
- Dosage can be hard to do.
- It's a distinct "heavy" than smoking.

Dosage: Consult your doctor before taking a drink of marijuana. Start with a little swallow and wait an hour before choosing whether or not to drink more.

Dabbing Medical Marijuana

How It Operates: a "dab" is a marijuana concentrate (hash oil, budder, tear, wax, etc.) that you warm up to elevated temperatures and inhale. Delivery systems differ but tend to be complicated and generally require the use of a butane torch. Concentrates may also comprise as much as 90% THC so that you will get a very elevated dose of psychoactive compounds.

This technique is not suggested for clients with poor THC tolerance or fresh to cannabis medicines!

Pros

- Useful for emergency medications for chronic diseases.
- Cost-efficient for clients in need of high-THC.
- Provides immediate relief.
- Concentrates are at a greater danger of carrying damaging chemicals.
- Solvents are used to remove medicinal chemicals, which may not be extracted correctly.
- It may trigger overdose, even if it is never deadly, but it can be very unpleasant and awkward.
- Devices are hard to use; accidental burns are more probable to occur.

Dosage: Consult your physician before you try to do, so it's likely more than you need. If you choose to attempt it, begin with just one 'tiny' hit, but understand it's going to have highly powerful psychoactive effects.

CONCENTRATES AND EXTRACTS

Concentrates let you experience cannabis in a variety of respects; they come in a variety of textures and can be used in a variety of respects. The look and feel of a focus do not necessarily imply its amount of quality (impacts, taste, potency); these are merely aesthetics that can assist you to stay track of your individual choices.

One of the main advantages of concentrates is the fast initiation moment and the capacity to produce a higher potency than cannabis flower consumption. Concentrates have a high bioavailability, which means that the effects you feel and experience, as well as the rate of absorption into your body, occur almost immediately. The impacts of a cannabis concentrate can last anywhere from 1 to 3 hours based on the person

What There Concentrates And Extracts?

Distillate

Concentrates come in many and contain the most desirable components of something. Orange juice focus, for instance, has the smell and flavor of orange fruit, but without surplus liquid, peel or paste. The same applies to the marijuana crop: aromas, flavorings, and other desirable components may be maintained while the leaves, roots, and other unwanted products are removed.

Extracts are a particular form of concentrate that uses solvents to extract the required crop, flower, or fruit components. For instance, vanilla extract is made by using alcohol as a solvent to remove the necessary flavor element, vanilla, from vanilla bean seeds.

The cannabis plant has complicated compounds or chemical components that can be used in a wide range of products. These compounds influence the appearance, taste, taste, and texture of cannabis products, as well as the physiological or psychoactive effects (if any) of cannabis products. The most desirable cannabis compounds are discovered in tiny, glittering constructions called trichomes throughout the cannabis plant. Cannabis concentrate relates to any item produced by the accumulation of trichomes from the plant.

Trichome Covered Cannabis

These frosty appendages cover the entire surface of the plant, particularly the flower buds. Trichomes comprise all cannabinoids (THC, CBD, etc.) and terpenes that offer distinct cultivars or types of cannabis their distinctive aromas and physical impacts.

Compared to the raw plant form of marijuana, cannabis concentrates give a higher potency, the faster start of the action and a wider variety of techniques of consumption. Depending on your preferences for use and the level of tolerance, the ideal dose may vary widely from person to person and even product to product.

Cannabis shake vape brownie balm Cannabis concentrates are varied and are used in a broad spectrum of products. With a choice of choices, you can fine-tune your cannabis experience and discover the perfect mix of cannabinoids and terpenes that appeals to your liking and gives you the most advantage.

Is There Any Distinction Between The Focus And The Extract?

All components are concentrated, but not all concentrates are liquids. While these words are used interchangeably, the main distinction between the gel and the sample is how trichomes are gathered. Extracts are a sort of concentrate produced using solvents (alcohol, carbon dioxide, etc.) that fundamentally wipe off the cannabis plant. Concentrates generated without the use of solutions are created using mechanical or physical means to extract and collect trichomes.

Butane Hash Oil (BHO), Rick Simpson Oil (RSO) and CO2-extracted cannabis wax are instances of products, each of which occurs in different textures such as shake, worse, budder and crumble. Various excerpts and compositions may give rise to different experiences from one item to another.

Rosin, dry sift, and kief is instances of concentrates that are produced without solvents.

Reduced-Fat Homogenized Ultra-Pasteurized

Milk" is also regarded as "2 percent milk," but this may sound confusing until you are acquainted with the item and its name. Once you get acquainted with the terminology used with concentrates, the more relaxed you will feel when checking the descriptions and marks. The names of the products may seem complicated. For instance, an item called "Hardcore OG Nug Run Shatter" may sound awkward. What does each of these phrases imply by that?

Producers and producers use particular terms and sentences to assist you in defining the main features, and features of cannabis concentrate. Certain conditions may be used on labels and descriptions of concentrated products to identify: the sort of cannabis plant material used to create focus The handling techniques The resulting textures The desired consumption methods

Input Materials Everything begins with cannabis plant material. The flower buds, leaves, and roots of the cannabis plant are jointly referred to as the beginning of the input material. The input material may change the subsequent cannabinoid and terpene profile of the cannabis focus. Also, the type or grade of the input material influences the potency and flavor of the subsequent concentrates.

Process Type

Cannabis concentrates are products produced by the accumulation of trichomes (a gland that produces cannabinoids and terpenes). There are several methods to distinguish the trichomes from the starting material. To create a focus, each of these procedures requires its specialized equipment and physical behavior or techniques.

Consistencies

Once cannabinoids and terpenes have been removed from the plant material, the resulting solution can take a variety of forms. These types enable nurses and customers to choose and choose the desired texture of the concentrated item; they are not necessarily an indication of how the concentrate tastes or affects the person.

Concentrates are secure, yet powerful. To eat a cannabis focus securely and efficiently, you must have a particular configuration with the suitable facilities to correctly trigger the focused cannabinoids And terpenes, too. When building the ideal dab rig, a fair amount of thought should be given to the components. Some customers, for instance, prefer to dab their titanium nail concentrates, while others may opt for quartz nails or bangers. Although quartz is less resistant than titanium, it heats up much quicker than titanium and provides a richer flavor. Depending on the pin of the banger, the majority of the users will heat it for about 30 seconds or until the banger starts to show a hot orange or red glow. Dabbing equipment From left: carbohydrate cap, quartz banger, titanium nail, dabber with carbohydrate cap, dab rig with quartz banger Textures And Consistency Terms such as shatter, worse, crumble, sugar, oil and sauce refer to the appearance of the concentrate (texture, color, and gravy) In other words, these conditions merely tell us about the look and feel of the focus. For instance, a focused item with the title informs you three stuff: the cannabis plant code used was "Blue Dream "Nug Run" indicates that the plant material used to make the extract was dried and cured flower The extract has a "shatter"-like consistency and texture The following seven terms describe the most common concentrated compositions found in.

Crumble Shatter are renowned for their fragile, glass-like texture. It could also have a snap-and-pull consistency. (Imagine a taffy candy that was drawn close before snapping). Shatters generally have a golden yellow to light amber color.

Budder is both oilier and weaker in texture. (Think of a butter or cake stick.) They're malleable, simple to manage, and they're sun-yellow to vivid orange. The butter-like texture enables the powder to be readily used as a spread on blunts or joints or to be stabbed using a dab device.

Crumble is a fragile variant of a budder or a worse. It has a crumbly-like honeycomb texture, as the name indicates. The color appears to be comparable to budder or worse, but instead of getting a shiny surface, it seems to have a matt shade of yellow.

Sugar, Sauce, and Crystalline Sugar is a word used for any concentrate that is comparable in texture to moist, sappy sugar. They are not uniform in design and usually have colors varying from a light yellow to deep amber.

The sauce is more substantial, more viscous in texture, and feels more sticky. The color of the sauce can vary from deep amber to light mustard. The sauce is comparable in texture and color to sugar but has a more standardized and prominent crystalline structure.

Crystalline is a single crystalline compound. As the name implies, THCa and CBD crystals are white crystals that can vary in density and size from small rocks to powders.

Smoking Methods

Cannabis focus can be eaten in a multitude of forms, either by sprinkling it on a tray or by bringing it to the joint for added potency or by spraying it with a dab tool or a mobile vape pen. The optimal technique of consumption relies on the sort and texture of the concentrate chosen, as well as on the private behaviors of the consumer. First, consider the instruments you have at your disposal and the composition of the focus when choosing which technique will function best. You might have seen excerpts like crushed and worse and wondered how best to smoke them? These components are malleable and straightforward to use in a dab system, while powdery concentrates, such as kief and crumble, can readily be liked by adding them to a more stable base like a flower. Here are some of the most popular techniques of smoking or spraying concentrates.

Topping Your Flower

Adding powdered jaw to your jar or winding wax around the joint is the most cost-effective way to use cannabis concentrates. These techniques do not involve any of the costly instruments needed to dab oil while improving the potency of your smoke and adding additional flavor to the mixture.

Tax and Cannabis Concentrate on Bowl From left: Bowl packed with flower topped with crumble, Twax with glass mouthpiece Dabbing The most common manner to eat cannabis concentrates is by spraying the focus using a dab system. This technique comprises of boiling the "wedge" (produced of either plastic, metal or metal) and then adding the concentrate straight to the warm ground. While there are many cheap methods to turn any water pipe into a dab rig, below is a list of products that you will need for a dab rig: from right: torch, dabber and carb cap combination with dab at the bottom, dab rig with quartz banger Vaporizers Vaping is the most subtle and affordable way to consume cannabis concentrates. The most prevalent type of vaping is a pre-filled cartridge that is attached to the battery. The round includes a heating element that goes into touch with the battery and heats the concentrate when it is enabled. This mixture of cells and cartridges is jointly referred to as a vape pen. Standard vape devices are powered by clicking a button or, in the event of a buttonless pen, merely dragging the cartridge from the mouthpiece. These pre-filled cartridges are not rechargeable and must be discarded after the concentrate has run out, but the battery can be saved and reused many times.

Handheld Vaporizer If you want to understand how to use cannabis oil in a more subtle and mobile manner, consider using a handheld vaporizer. With a vaporizer, you can directly fill the cabinet with any focus and connect the box to the battery. Typically, the cell includes a heating coil that transforms the concentrate into a vapor when the customer pushes a key. Unlike a dab facility, this technique does not involve any extra facilities, but still provides you the capacity to pre-film the chamber with any focus and use it on request.

What Is The Man Extraction Types?

If you want to know how to create THC oil or other types of cannabis concentrate, there are two methods to do this: physically Separating trichome or using liquid solvents from the plant.

Physical Segregation

During the physical separation process, trichome cells are separated from cannabis beginning material by physical intervention, such as squeezing or pushing. Think of the trichome cells as the fruit of the lemon tree: physical division is comparable to the cracking of the citrus tree to remove the nut.

For example, when dry sifting, cannabis is shaken through a series of screens in specific sizes to ensure that only the trichome heads pass through to the final product. Rosin is produced using a focused mixture of heat and strain to force the required compounds out of the plant. The main idea of physical segregation is that immediate physical activity outcomes in the manifestation of trichomes.

Liquid Solvent Extraction

All solvent extractions use the same fundamental workflow: a liquid solvent is used to divide the active compounds from the trichome gland to produce a solution. This solution must be further developed until nothing is left but the required compounds.

Cannabis oils concentrate and extract all act as umbrella conditions under which distinct products are stored: steam oil, hash, tinctures, dabs, CBD oil, and any other item dreamed of by cannabis chemists.

An oil, focus, or extract is any material obtained from a cannabis flower that is handled in a focused shape, but each type of cannabis oil is distinctive.

But why bother with the concentrates when you've tried a real bud? Flower may be good enough for you, but there are many reasons to explore the many options and medicines offered in the form of extracts: you don't have to smoke extracts. Most customers choose to spray or ingest concentrates at a smoke-free dose.

Cannabis oils are beneficial. It requires less item to have the necessary knowledge.

Extracts have been refined. Essential oils and cannabinoids are removed from plant material to produce a soft, clean inhalation when vaporized Gone is the day when cannabis was used to smoke flowers or to infuse them into home-made edible products. Nowadays, cannabis users have more decisions than ever before because of the ever-expanding globe of marijuana concentrates and extracts.

These products come in a multitude of distinct types, but the thing they all share in common is their incredible power. Although the terms "cannabis concentrate" and "cannabis extract" are often used interchangeably, they are not the same thing and to be precise, and it is essential to know the difference between them.

Weed Concentrates

The universe of marijuana concentrates and extracts provides a wide range of consumer choices.

The Difference Between Marijuana Concentrates vs. Extracts

The Oxford Learner's Dictionary defines the noun "concentrate" as "a substance that is made stronger because water or other substances have been removed." This is true of cannabis concentrates they're much stronger than regular cannabis flower.

When it comes to marijuana, "concentrates" is an umbrella term that also includes all extracts. This means that while all cannabis extracts are concentrates, not all cannabis concentrates can be considered extracts.

Why is this? A marijuana concentrate uses mechanical methods to collect the plant's trichomes (which are packed with cannabinoids such as THC and CBD). Meanwhile, a marijuana extract takes the added step of using some solvent to strip the trichomes away from the plant material.

Using this necessary explanation to lay out the difference between concentrates and cannabis extracts, the hash would be considered a focus, as it uses mechanical methods (sifting through screens or even bubble bags) to remove trichomes. Meanwhile, BHO wax is a concentrate, but specifically, it's an extract (because manufacturers use butane to extract the desired cannabinoids and terpenes).

Different Types Of Marijuana Concentrates

Over the years, cannabis consumers have developed a wide variety of concentrates that are used by medical patients to get a more carefully-controlled (or stronger) dose, as well as recreational consumers looking for exciting and intense new ways to enjoy their favorite herb. Here are some of the most common cannabis concentrates and extracts, how they're made, and how they're typically consumed.

Butane Hash Oil (BHO)

Butane hash oil (often referred to as BHO or butane honey oil), is an umbrella term for several different concentrates (including shatter, wax, crumble, etc.). Butane hash oil is a marijuana extract that's made by forcing butane through plant material. After the extraction process is complete, the resulting substance contains no plant material just high percentages of the cannabinoids and terpenes that give cannabis its effects, taste, and flavor.

Forms Of BHO

Depending on how BHO is handled, it will either remain in an oil form or harden into one of its other ways.

The different forms of BHO include:

Sap: soft and oozy, but not as runny as oil.

Wax: one of the most common forms of BHO available on the market, the wax is solid but soft and pliable.

Crumble: A bit harder than wax, crumble easily breaks apart when handled.

Budder: a whipped, highly pure, and rare form of BHO, budder has the smooth consistency of butter.

Pull and snap: BHO that can be pulled and caught into smaller pieces (similar to taffy).

Shatter: BHO in its hardest form, shatter takes on the consistency of glass. Next, to wax, this is one of the most widely available types of BHO.

Concentrate Weed BHO

Butane hash oil (BHO) is a cannabis extract that can take many forms – from runny oil to glasslike shatter.

Consuming BHO

One of the biggest questions people have when dealing with different types of marijuana concentrates for the first time is how to destroy them. As BHO is so different in appearance from traditional marijuana flower, it's common for novice consumers to end up with a bit of shatter or wax and have no idea what to do with it.

Proper consumption of BHO requires a dab rig or a vaporizer that's specially-designed for cannabis concentrates. A dab rig is a bong-like device that's fitted with a "nail" or a "banger a piece of metal or glass that's heated to high temperatures to vaporize the concentrate. Some rigs require the use of a handheld torch to generate these high temperatures, while others have "e-nails" or electronic nails that can be plugged in to be heated. This process is known as "dabbing," and the BHO that gets vaporized are commonly referred to as "dabs."

There are also particular vaporizers from larger desktop models to portable vape pens that are made for dabbing. Not just any vaporizer will do; however; it's essential to use a model that's specially designed to handle these kinds of cannabis concentrates. Failure to do so will result in an oily mess and will likely damage the vaporizer.

BHO can be found as a high THC concentrate or a CBD concentrate, depending on the strain it's extracted from.

Live Resin

Live resin is a type of BHO that many consider being the "champagne" of cannabis concentrates. Highly sought-after, it perfectly preserves the terpenes and flavor profiles of the cannabis strain from which it's extracted.

This happens when manufacturers flash-freeze cannabis plants mere minutes after they're harvested, rather than curing them (as is done with the plant material used for most BHO products). The result is an aromatic, flavorful marijuana extract with a robust terpene profile and potent levels of cannabinoids. This concentrate is consumed just like any BHO product with a dab rig or vaporizer.

Live resin that's properly manufactured will feature a balanced amount of crystals (created when the THC is extracted) and liquid (the terpene extract). It will range in color from a beautiful light gold to a warm amber tone. Because of the extra care that's taken in the processing of live resin, it's one of the most expensive cannabis extracts.

Every cannabis plant is covered in trichomes. These tiny, resinous glands contain the cannabinoids that give marijuana and even hemp the effects that make them so valuable to medical and recreational consumers. When these trichomes dry and fall off, they're known as kief, and they're one of the oldest kinds of cannabis concentrate.

Weed Extracts Kief

One of the oldest cannabis concentrates, kief is the trichomes or marijuana pollen that fall off of the flower when it's ground or handled.

Harvesting Kief

Kief can be harvested as a by-product of marijuana flower by collecting it in the bottom of a four-piece herb grinder. It can also be managed more directly by various means. The dried herb can be placed on silk screens and manipulated or pounded, forcing the pollen to fall into a bowl or collection tray beneath. The collected kief can then be pressed into hashish potent discs or balls of sticky marijuana pollen. Flower can also be wrapped inside filter bags and placed in ice water. This process freezes the trichomes and breaks them off of the plant material, and it's how bubble hash is made.

Consuming Kief/Hashish

The consumption of kief or compressed hashish doesn't involve any specialized equipment. Some people break up hash or sprinkle kief inside marijuana or tobacco cigarettes. They can also be smoked in pipes or bongs.

Kief can also be used to create marijuana-infused edibles. To activate the cannabinoids and enjoy their effects, however, it's essential to decarboxylate the kief first. This involves heating it many people spread it on an oven-safe dish or baking sheet and put it in a 250-degree oven for about 20 minutes. Once it's decarboxylated, kief can be mixed into tea, hot chocolate, baked goods, or other edibles.

Cannabis Moon Rocks

If the live resin is the champagne of the cannabis world, then moon rocks are its caviar. Cannabis moon rocks combine traditional marijuana buds with two types of marijuana concentrates: BHO and kief. Specifically, moon rocks involve dipping a marijuana bud into BHO before rolling it in kief. When moon rocks were first developed, people used the Girl Scout Cookies strain to make them, but fans of this type of cannabis concentrate can handle any pressure they prefer. Treating marijuana buds in this way can nearly double the amount of THC in them, creating potent nuggets that can run as high as 50 to 64 percent THC.

Consuming Moon Rocks

Moon rocks can be broken up and smoked in a pipe, a bong, or a bubbler. They can also be distributed throughout a joint. Because they're coated in kief, consumers should take care when handling them. It's important to avoid grinding moon rocks in a dry herb grinder, as this will result in loss of the kief.

Weed Concentrate

Known as the caviar of cannabis concentrates, moon rocks are marijuana nuggets coated in butane honey oil before being rolled in kief.

Cannabis Oil/Rick Simpson Oil

Cannabis oil is a cannabis extract created by using a solvent to form a cannabinoid-rich oil. Depending on whether the oil is made using hemp or marijuana (and depending on the marijuana strain used), cannabis oil can be extremely rich in THC, high in CBD, or have a balance of both.

Rick Simpson Oil (also known as RSO or Phoenix Tears) is full-full-spectrum cannabis oil, meaning that it contains a wide range of terpenes and cannabinoids that include THC as well as CBD. It was created by Rick Simpson, a Canadian engineer who designed the concoction to cure his skin cancer. He began sharing his recipe with the public and gave his oil away for free for some time before being arrested and targeted by Canadian law enforcement.

Today, Simpson lives in Europe, but he still promotes the effectiveness of his oil recipe, which is made by soaking cannabis plant material in ethanol, butane, or another solvent to extract the cannabinoids. Many versions of "Rick Simpson Oil" are available online, but Simpson maintains that he has no association with any of these products and encourages consumers to make their own if possible.

Consuming Cannabis Oil/Rick Simpson Oil

Cannabis oil and RSO make excellent alternatives to smoking marijuana flower – particularly for medical consumers who need a potent, carefully-controlled dose of THC or CBD. The oils can be taken orally in a variety of ways. Some people use a syringe to place a small amount directly in the mouth. Specific amounts can be dosed out and taken in capsules. Cannabis oils can be mixed into coffee, tea, smoothies, or other edibles. Many people (such as Simpson) also use them topically.

Cannabis oil must be decarboxylated to maximize its potency. This means bringing it to a temperature of 230 degrees Fahrenheit either in an oven or using a coffee or candle warmer. Small, pin-prick-sized bubbles on the surface of the oil are an indication that decarboxylation is happening; once this activity ceases, the process is complete.

Cannabis Tinctures

While cannabis oil is an extraction that (as its name implies) is in oil form, cannabis tinctures use alcohol extraction to create a cannabinoid-filled liquid. In the early 20th century, cannabis tinctures were a popular form of medication. Today, people are rediscovering the medical benefits of taking advantage of THC and CBD in concentrated and carefully-controlled doses.

Consuming Cannabis Tinctures

Tinctures may be applied by placing a few drops or sprays under the tongue. Taking cannabis concentrates in sublingual tincture form works faster than consuming cannabis edibles because the tinctures don't have to pass through the digestive tract.

Concentrate Weed Tincture

Tinctures are marijuana extracts that can be applied as a spray or drops under the tongue.

The Effect Of Cannabis Extracts And Concentrates

As the dictionary definition states, concentrates are stronger than the non-concentrated substance. This means that marijuana extracts and concentrates are much more potent than traditional cannabis flower.

THC Concentrate Effects

How strong? It depends on the concentrate. Marijuana flower contains various amounts of THC, ranging from less than 10 percent to well over 20 percent. Kief can contain as much as 70 percent THC. Meanwhile, butane hash oil (BHO) concentrates can hold from 60 to 90 percent THC.

The effect of THC concentrates will be a powerful version of what one would experience from consuming traditional marijuana flower that contains THC. Intense euphoria, dry mouth, increased appetite, visual trails, couch lock, and an intensified auditory sense are universal. In those with a low tolerance to THC, an elevated heart rate, anxiety, and paranoia are possible.

CBD Concentrate Effects

Hemp can also be used to make concentrates. Hemp flower contains around 3.5 percent CBD, while oil extracted from hemp might hold up to 20 percent CBD. Meanwhile, CBD isolate can contain as much as 99 percent CBD.

Similar to THC concentrates, the effects of consuming CBD concentrates are the same as consuming marijuana or hemp flower that contains lesser amounts of CBD the effects are intensified. Many people experience a sense of relaxation and well-being of CBD concentrates. At high doses, dry mouth and lightheadedness can occur.

Medical Use Of Cannabis Concentrates

The medical uses for cannabis concentrates vary as widely as the types of concentrates themselves. Because concentrates come in many different forms and strengths and are derived from different marijuana strains (as well as hemp), they contain wildly different cannabinoid and terpene profiles. This makes them useful for a whole host of medical conditions and ailments. Here are a few of the most common reasons medical patients turn to cannabis concentrates for relief:

Pain

Both THC and CBD are excellent at relieving pain, which is why people who are dealing with severe or chronic pain often look to marijuana concentrates or hemp-derived cannabis extracts to get relief.

Nausea

THC is also an active anti-nausea agent and one that's frequently used by cancer patients who are dealing with chemotherapy-related nausea. Because it also stimulates appetite and quells pain, THC can help address multiple issues that cancer patients frequently face when undergoing treatment for the disease.

Anxiety

While THC can exacerbate anxiety in those who are prone to it, studies have shown that CBD has the opposite effect. Not only can CBD calm anxiety; it can help counteract some of the anxiety-inducing effects of THC for patients who need to dose with THC for medical purposes.

Cancer

For years, patients have used cannabis and its concentrates to treat symptoms of the disease as well as effects from chemotherapy and radiation. Scientists have also begun to study marijuana as a potential cancer treatment, and while those studies have been promising, they haven't yet been transformed into a real-world treatment. People like Rick Simpson feel that the reviews are enough and use cannabis oil as a curative, rather than a symptomatic treatment.

Weed Concentrates Cannabis Oil

Concentrates such as cannabis oil are used for a whole host of medical conditions and ailments.

Cannabis Concentrates Concerns And Controversy

While cannabis concentrates such as kief and hash have been consumed for centuries, extracts don't come without some degree of controversy. This is in portion due to concerns over the manufacturing process involved with extracts such as BHO, as well as the strength of marijuana concentrates.

At-Home BHO Manufacturing

In recent years, the headlines have been filled with stories of at-home BHO manufacturing gone awry. Because the process involves butane, a highly flammable solvent, people who lack the proper equipment or know-how can easily ignite a fire or worse. In January 2019, two California men were arrested after the home in which they were making BHO exploded. While BHO is sold in various legal cannabis dispensaries, those types of products are manufactured in carefully-controlled laboratory settings. Some manufacturers use carbon dioxide as a safer alternative to explosive butane.

Potency Of Cannabis Concentrates

Another concern with marijuana extracts and concentrates is their potency. Unlike smoking marijuana flower, which allows consumers to enjoy a puff and experience a relatively small amount of THC, concentrates pack a huge THC punch – especially for those who are inexperienced with marijuana.

Because BHO wax and shatter are available at many legal dispensaries, this means that they can be easily purchased by novice concentrate consumers. If they aren't properly educated by a knowledgeable budtender or friend, it's easy to overdo these kinds of extracts.

Dabs aren't the only kind of marijuana extract that holds the potential for overconsumption. While cannabis oils make it easy for consumers to control their dose carefully, this is only the case if the oils are clearly labeled to educate people about how much to ingest. If a label is too complicated, doesn't feature proper dosing information, or is ignored, it's easy for consumers to overconsume cannabis oil.

Weed Concentrates Dabbing

Dabbing concentrates like wax and shatters leads to more intense effects than smoking marijuana flower.

Knowledge Is Power With Cannabis Concentrates

Cannabis concentrates and extracts offer a whole new world of choices to consumers both those who enjoy marijuana recreationally and are looking for exciting new ways to ingest it as well as medical marijuana patients who need doses that are more powerful and precise than they can get from marijuana flower. Marijuana extracts and concentrates provide a massive variety of options, whether an individual would like to relax and smoke a bit of hashish, experience the intense high brought on by dabbing, or use cannabis oil topically to treat a medical condition.

The important thing for consumers to remember with marijuana concentrates is to start low and slow. This means that novices should begin with the lowest dosage possible and wait a while before trying more. While dabbing wax or shatter produces a high in a matter of minutes, drinking a kief-infused cup of hot chocolate could take an hour or more to generate effects. By remembering "low and slow," consumers raise the chances of their experience being a positive, rather than an uncomfortable one.

MEDICAL APPLICATION OF CBD

The potential health benefits of CBD, how it can be used, potential risks and problems related to its legality in the United States The National Food and Drug Administration (FDA) has endorsed the prescription of Epidiolex, a purified type of CBD oil, for the treatment of two types of epilepsy.

CBD is one of the many compounds known as cannabinoids in the cannabis plant. Researchers looked at the possible therapeutic uses of CBD.CBD oils are oils containing levels of CBD. The standards and utilizes such oils differ.

Is It CBD Marijuana?

CBD oil may have several wellness advantages for CBD oil. Until lately, the most famous cannabis compound was delta-9 tetrahydrocannabinol (THC). This is the most active ingredient in marijuana. Marijuana includes both THC and CBD, which have distinct impacts.

THC produces a mind-altering "high" when an individual smokes it or utilizes it to cook. This is because THC breaks down when we add heat and put it in the body.

It's a distinct CDB. Unlike THC, it's not psychoactive. These imply that the CBD does not alter the state of mind of a person when they use it.

CBD does, however, appear to generate essential modifications in the body, and some study indicates that it has medical advantages.

Where Is The CBD Coming From?

The CDB originates from the cannabis plant. Folks seek advice from cannabis crops as either hemp or marijuana, supported their consciousness-altering drug levels. Hemp crops legal below the measure should comprise but zero.3 percent of consciousness-altering drug.

Over the years, marijuana breeders have by selection bred their crops to contain elevated concentrations of consciousness-altering drug and alternative compounds that were of interest to them, actually because the compounds generated a smell or had a special impact on the flowers of the plant. However, hemp producers have scarcely created changes to the plant. These hemp crops square measure used for the assembly of CBD oil.

All cannabinoids, together with CBD, have impacts on the body by attaching to bound receptors. Some cannabinoids square measure generated on their own by the figure. It additionally has two cannabinoid receptors referred to as CB1 and CB2 receptors.CB1 receptors square measure gift throughout the body; however, there square measure several within the brain.

CB1 receptors within the brain act with balance and motion, pain, feelings, and mood, thinking, desire, and memory, and alternative tasks. The consciousness-altering drug is connected to the receptors.

CB2 receptors square measure additional common within the system. Inflammation and pain are influenced. Researchers once believed that CBD was coupled to those CB2 receptors, however currently it seems that CBD isn't directly coupled to either receptor.

Instead, the body seems to be directed to use additional of its cannabinoids.

CBD advantages will affect an individual's health in an exceeding multitude of respects.

Natural pain relief and anti-inflammatory properties folks tend to use prescription or over-the-counter medicines to alleviate stiffness and pain, together with chronic pain. Some people suppose that CBD may be an additional natural possibility.

Authors of a groundwork discharged within the Journal of Experimental medication discovered that CBD had significantly slashed chronic inflammation and pain in some mice and rats, too. Researchers instructed that non-psychoactive compounds in marijuana, like CBD, could give new treatment for chronic pain. Quitting smoking and drug withdrawals Some no-hit proof indicates that CBD use will assist people in stopping smoking.

A pilot analysis discharged in addictive Behaviors discovered that smokers United Nations agency used CBD-containing inhalers preserved fewer cigarettes than traditional and had no alternative cravings for vasoconstrictive. A comparable study, discharged in Neurotherapeutics, discovered that CBD might well be a no-hit medical aid for people with opioid addiction diseases. Researchers have noted that CBD has reduced the number of illnesses related to substance use disorders. They enclosed anxiety, indications of mood, pain, and sleep disorder. Additional studies square measure needed. However, these findings recommend that CBD could facilitate stop or scale back withdrawal symptoms.

Epilepsy when researching the protection and efficaciousness of CBD oil within the medical aid of encephalopathy, the Food and Drug Administration supported the utilization of CBD (Epidiolex) as a therapeutic aid for two uncommon convulsion things in 2018.

In the U.S., a doctor could order Epidiolex for the medical aid of: Lennox-Gastaut Syndrome (LGS), a malady that happens between the ages of three and five years and involves totally different forms of Dravet Syndrome (DS) seizures, AN uncommon genetic condition that occurs within the initial year of life and affects periodic, fever-related seizures. The Food and Drug Administration claimed that doctors couldn't order Epidiolex for kids aged than two years of era. The proper dose shall be determined by the medico or druggist on the grounds of weight. Alternative medical specialty signs and disturbances Researchers square measure investigation the impacts of CBD on totally different medical disorders.

Findings projected that CBD might also cure several epilepsy-related issues like neurodegeneration, neural injury, and medical disorders.

Another analysis, discharged in Current Pharmaceutical style, discovered that CBD would generate impacts such as those of bound antipsychotic drug medicine which the compound will give secure and economical medical aid for people with dementia praecox. An additional study, however, is needed cancer control. Some scientists have discovered that CBD can demonstrate to be in the fight against cancer. Authors of a study released in the British Journal of Clinical Pharmacology have found proof that CBD has substantially helped avoid the spread of disease. Researchers also observed that the compound tends to inhibit the development and destruction of cancer cells. They noted out that CBD has a low level of toxicity. They called for further studies on its ability to accompany conventional cancer treatments.

Anxiety Disorders

Doctors often recommend individuals with acute anxiety to prevent cannabis because THC can cause or amplify emotions of anxiety and paranoia.

However, the writers of the Neurotherapeutics assessment discovered that CBD could assist in decreasing anxiety in individuals with certain associated illnesses.

According to the assessment, CBD may reduce anxiety-related behaviors in people with conditions such as post-traumatic stress disorder overall anxiety disorder panic disorder personal anxiety disorder obsessive-compulsive disorder Current medications for these diseases may add to new infections and side effects that may lead some people to stop taking them. No further definite proof presently connects CBD to adverse effects, and the writers called for new research of the compound as an anxiety therapy.

Type 1 diabetes

Type 1 is caused by inflammation that happens when the immune system assaults pancreatic cells. Clinical hemorheology and microcirculation have shown that CBD can relieve this inflammation of the pancreas. This may be the first stage of the discovery of CBD-based type 1 diabetes treatment.

A report presented that same year in Lisbon, Portugal, suggested that CBD could reduce inflammation and protect against or stop the development of type 1 diabetes.

Acne

Acne treatment is another practical use of CBD. The disease is due, in part, to inflammation and overworked sebaceous glands in the body.

Journal of Clinical Investigation found that CBD helps decrease the production of sebum that adds to acne, partly owing to its anti-inflammatory effect on the body. Sebum is an oily substance, and overproduction may contribute to acne.

CBD can be a prospective treatment for acne vulgaris, the most common form of acne.

Alzheimer's Disease

The initial research published in the Journal of Alzheimer's Disease found that CBD was able to prevent an increase in the lack of social recognition among participants. This implies that CBD could assist individuals in the early phases of Alzheimer's still can identify the faces of individuals they understand.

These are the first proof that CBD may slow down the development of Alzheimer's disease

Legality

Marijuana leaves CBD oil is a cannabis-based cannabinoid.

The present legality of CBD is hazy. Hemp and hemp products are legal under the Farm Bill, as long as their THC content is less than 0.3 percent.

However, there is still some uncertainty about the specifics.

People should inspect the legislation of their own country and any travel destination. They should bear in mind that the FDA has not yet authorized any non-prescription products.

Recent advances: CBD Epilepsy Oil FDA has endorsed the use of CBD to treat two kinds of epilepsy.

"Today, the ГDA has endorsed a purified type of drug cannabidiol (CBD) that is one of more than 80 effective substances in marijuana. The fresh item has been accepted for the treatment of seizures connected with two unusual, serious types of epilepsy in clients two years of era and older." The FDA has not endorsed the use of marijuana or all of its parts.

The organization has only endorsed a purified variant of one CBD drug for a specific therapeutic intent.

The choice to approve the item was based on the outcomes of a sound clinical trial.

Patients will obtain medicine in a secure dosage.

Side Effects

Many small trials have looked at the safety of CBD in adolescents. They found that adolescents tend to tolerate a wide variety of doses.

Researchers discovered that there were no critical side effects on the central nervous system, vital signs, or mood, even among individuals who used elevated doses.

Fatness is the most common side effect. Some individuals also report diarrhea and shifts in their appetite or weight.

However, individuals need to talk to their doctor before taking a CBD course. The drug may communicate with some over-the-counter (OTC) aids, dietary supplements, and CBD prescription drugs, particularly those that caution against the use Its grapefruit.

CBD may also interfere with the enzyme called the P450 cytochrome complex. This may influence the capacity of the liver to break down toxins and increase the likelihood of liver toxicity.

Risks There is still an absence of accessible information on long-term safety.

Also, to date, scientists have not conducted research concerning kids.

Side Effects Of Epidiolex

As far as the product approved by the FDA for the therapy of two types of epilepsy is concerned, the following adverse effects have been observed in clinical studies: signs of liver issues associated with the central nervous system, such as irritability and lethargy, decreased gastrointestinal appetite issues. And other sensitivity reactions reduced urination breathing. It is essential to monitor anyone who uses this drug for indications of a mood shift.

Research indicates that it is probable that an individual getting the item will become addicted.

Side effects of other forms of CBD There is often an absence of proof as to the safety of fresh or alternative therapy choices. Usually, scientists have not carried out the complete range of experiments.

Anyone who is considering using CBD should speak to a skilled healthcare professional in advance.

The FDA only authorized CBD for the therapy of two unusual and severe types of epilepsy.

If drugs do not have FDA approval, it may be hard to understand whether an item includes a secure or efficient amount of CBD.

Unapproved products may not have the characteristics or contents indicated on the package.

It is essential to remember that during pregnancy, scientists have related marijuana use to impaired neuron fetal development. Regular use among adolescents is correlated with problems related to memory, conduct, and intellect.

How to use CBD is one of the compounds in marijuana CBD is only one of the potential compounds in marijuana and is not psychoactive. Smoking cannabis isn't the same thing as using CBD oil.

Using CBD oil is not the same as using or smoking whole cannabis.= An individual can use CBD oil in a variety of forms to relieve multiple problems.

If it is prescribed by a doctor to manage LGS or DS, it is essential to follow their directions.

CBD-based products come in a variety of types. Some may be various with separate ingredients or beverages or done with a pipette or a dropper.

Others are available in capsules or as a thick paste to be massaged in the skin. Some goods are available as sprays for use under the thumb. Recommended dosages differ between individuals and rely on variables such as body weight, item concentration and safety issues Some people consider using CBD oil to assist treat: chronic pain epilepsy Parkinson's disease of Huntington's sleep disorders glaucoma Due to absence of FDA regulation for most CBD products, seek guidance from a medical professional prior to treatment.

As regulation rises in the United States, more particular dosages and prescriptions will begin to arise.

It is essential to compare distinct products of CBD oil after debating doses and hazards with a doctor and investigating local, regional legislation.

BONUS: 2 CANNABIS INFUSED EDIBLE RECIPES

Cannabis-Infused Honey Fennel Gingerbread

There's nothing like waking up to the smell of fresh gingerbread. Cozy up on the couch with your loved ones and a slice of warm cannabis-infused honey fennel gingerbread. This cannabis edible recipe is the perfect way to enjoy the holidays with company or your family.

This recipe makes a single 2-pound gingerbread cake.

Ingredients:

- 6 ounces canna-butter (see below)
- 1 cup water
- 1/4 cup olive oil
- 3/4 cup honey
- 1/4 cup milk
- 1/4 cup full-fat plain yogurt
- 2 large eggs, beaten
- 1 1/2 cup unbleached white flour
- 2 teaspoon ground ginger
- 1 teaspoon baking soda
- 1 teaspoon baking powder
- 1 tablespoon fresh grated ginger
- 2 teaspoon crushed fennel seed

Make canna-butter at least one day ahead of time:

Add water and one pound of butter to a saucepan and simmer at low heat. As the butter melts, add in 1 ounce of your decarboxylated ground marijuana.

Maintain low heat and let mixture simmer for 3-4 hours, stirring occasionally.

Pour cannabis-infused butter in airtight container and keep in the fridge to harden.

Instructions:

Preheat the oven to 325 degrees. Line an 8.5 x 4.5 inch loaf pan with parchment paper.

Place 6 ounces of cannabis-infused butter and honey in a medium saucepan on low heat until the butter is melted (you will have leftover butter that can be used later).

Remove from heat and add the olive oil, milk, yogurt, whisking until mixed. Place aside to cool.

In a medium-sized mixing bowl, whisk together the flour, ground ginger, baking powder, and baking soda.

Place the fennel seeds into a small skillet set at medium-low heat for a few minutes to toast. Transfer them to a cutting board and crush the seeds.

Add the crushed fennel, fresh ginger, and eggs to the honey mixture in the saucepan mix well.

Pour the honey mixture into the dry mix, one-third at a time, whisking gently between each addition.

Pour combined batter into loaf pan and spread out evenly. Place the loaf pan into the oven and bake for 50-60 minutes or until top is shiny and golden and inserted knife comes out clean.

Remove pan from heat and allow it to cool in the pan for about 15 minutes before placing it on a rack to cool another 30 minutes before slicing and serving.

Cannabis And Cranberry Stuffing

Stuffing is a staple in many homes during large family gatherings around the holidays. This rich, delicious holiday stuffing may take center stage at your next grown-up holiday get-together.

This marijuana edible recipe will make around 8 servings.

Ingredients:

- 1 loaf of white bread
- 1 pound of bacon
- 2-3 carrots
- 2 celery stalks
- 1/2 yellow onion
- 1/2 cup dried cranberries
- 1/2 cup canna-butter (see recipe above)
- 1 cup turkey, chicken or vegetable stock
- 4 tablespoons sage
- 4 tablespoons crushed unsalted cashews
- Salt and pepper to taste

Instructions:

Preheat oven to 375 degrees.

Cut bread into small cubes small dice vegetables.

Cook bacon in the frying pan until about ¾ of the way done. Add vegetables and cook until tender season with salt and pepper to taste.

Add cranberries, canna-butter, and stock to pan. Stir together and let simmer for 2-3 minutes.

Remove pan from heat. Add sage and cashews to the mixture and stir. In a large bowl, add bread squares and liquid mixture, being careful not to over mix. Add mixture to 9″ x 13″ baking pan — Place in the oven and bake for 25 minutes.

CONCLUSION

After assessing the effects, addictiveness, and their impacts, marijuana was classified as having a mild effect on businesses. Marijuana is produced from the dried, broken leaves, roots, seeds, and flowers of the hemp plant (Cannabis Saliva). It can come in many distinct, but the most frequent is the frozen leaves and the presence of long green leaves.

The short-term effects are not significant (sleepiness, absence of motor control, and reduced energy levels) and only last for a brief period of the moment (about two hours after the ingestion of the medication). Unfortunately, when marijuana is often used, long-term impacts start to occur, they are more severe and can last a lifetime. Long-term, smoked cannabis (the most common way of entering the bloodstream) can ruin the respiratory system, causing the person to develop chronic cough to increase significantly the likelihood of heart failure and cancer. In reality, marijuana smoke has a higher quantity of cancer-producing agents than tobacco smoke. Marijuana can also trigger brain damage when done frequently. Some signs include memory loss, brief attention span, and permanent sleepiness leading to job losses and academic defects. Marijuana is not very addictive (only 9 percent of users are addicted, but it doesn't seem to prevent individuals from taking it. Studies indicate that in 2010, of the approximately 7.1 million Americans categorized as addicted to or abused illicit drugs, almost 4.5 million were addicted to or abused marijuana. Drug withdrawal symptoms have a mild effect, such as increased cravings and sleeplessness.

Besides, we think that present strategies aimed at regulating the availability of marijuana should be severely reconsidered. The proven ineffectiveness of the command of use through the prohibition of production and the substantial expenses of applying such a strategy renders it very unlikely that any kind of partial prohibition strategy would be efficient in lowering marijuana use considerably below current rates. Besides, it seems likely that the removal of criminal sanctions will be given serious consideration by the federal government and the states in the foreseeable future. A range of alternative strategies should, therefore, be regarded.

At this time, the form of specific alternatives to current policies and their likely impact on patterns of use can not be determined with certainty. It is feasible that, after thorough research, all options will turn out to have so many disadvantages that none of them could force public consensus. However, to increase the probability of good legislation over the lengthy-term, further study should be performed on the biological, cognitive, developmental and cultural effects of marijuana use, on the composition and functioning of drug exchanges, and the relationship of different circumstances of accessibility to habits of consumption.